CONTENTS

Introduction:..Page 1

Chapter One: What is cancer?............................Page 5

All in the genes?...Page 6

So what causes cells to multiply out of control
and form a tumour?..Page 7

Just half an hour a day on your mobile could increase
your risk of brain cancer by up to 40%.............................Page 8

Could the medical profession have got it wrong?..............Page 9

Mainstream medicine's approach to fighting the disease.................Page 11

Chapter Two: Diet..Page 13

The disease-fighting nutrients that provide a vital defence
against cancer...Page 13

Healthy eating tips – your way to 5 a day.........................Page 13

What you don't eat is just as important as what you do eat.............Page 15

The anti-cancer rainbow diet..Page 16

Allicin..Page 17

A pungent reminder: garlic remains a potent player in the
fight against cancer...Page 17

Limonoids..Page 17

How the health benefits of oranges extend beyond vitamin C.........Page 18

Carotenoids..Page 18

How eating more spinach could reduce ovarian cancer risk.............Page 18

Catechins...Page 20

Green tea helps destroy breast cancer and oesophageal
cancer cells...Page 20

Chlorophyll..Page 22

Eat your dark leafy greens to ward off prostate cancer.........Page 22

Sulforaphane...Page 23

How a substance found in broccoli can slow the spread of
breast cancer by up to 90%!..Page 23

Lycopene..Page 24

Why tomatoes could protect you from prostate cancer.........Page 25

Ellagic acid..Page 25

Ellagic acid heralds a vital breakthrough in the prevention
of cancer...Page 25

Resveratrol...Page 26

Resveratrol showing promise in the fight against breast,
bowel and liver cancers..Page 27

Anthocyanins..Page 28

The secret of blueberry's 4-pronged attack on cancer..........Page 28

Why all good things come to those who wait......................Page 28

Why opting for organic produce is worth the extra pennies.....Page 29

New research findings suggest that reducing your calorie
intake by just 5% could lower your risk of cancer..............Page 32

More anti-cancer foods to add to your shopping list.............Page 33

Study findings uncover cancer-fighting properties
linked to avocados..Page 33

Researchers reveal how watercress plays a vital role in the
prevention of cancer..Page 34

Soya – boosting your intake could reduce your risk of
breast and prostate cancer...Page 36

The acrylamide and cancer link..Page 39

Rosemary is proving an important defence against cancer.....Page 39

Include more olive oil in your diet......................................Page 41

Mediterranean diet cuts breast cancer risk in older women.....Page 42

The Cancer Survival Manual

Tomorrow's Cancer Breakthroughs TODAY

By Rachael Linkie

 Agora Health Limited

If you have any queries, please contact Customer Services at: Agora Health Limited, 7th Floor, Sea Containers House, 20 Upper Ground, London SE1 9JD. You may also call 020 7633 3630 or send a fax to 020 7633 3740.

ISBN: 978-0-9560100-1-8

Why an apple a day could keep pancreatic cancer at bay.................Page 43

Could a curry offer effective protection against colon
and breast cancer?..Page 45

Oily fish can help cut colorectal cancer risk...................................Page 46

Eat more Brazil nuts to keep prostate and breast cancers at bay........Page 48

Vitamin B17 – the remarkable, secret nutrient that one
doctor claims can lead to "cancer cells dying off like flies!"............Page 49

How a unique form of honey can boost the immune
systems of cancer patients undergoing chemotherapy...................Page 52

Dietary advice that could lower your breast cancer risk.................Page 55

Water helps your body eliminate poisonous waste products.........Page 58

Follow these 7 steps to protect your health against
fluoride's harmful effects...Page 59

Chapter Three: Prostate Cancer...Page 61

Look out for these warning signs that can spell prostate trouble...Page 61

Could you be at risk?...Page 62

Time to test your prostate? You need to read this...........................Page 63

A PSA (prostatic specific antigen) blood test................................Page 63

Digital rectal examination (DRE)..Page 63

PSA test results can vary. Get tested twice!...................................Page 64

Additional tests that help detect prostate cancer...........................Page 65

New test for prostate cancer offers hope in the fight
against the disease..Page 66

What conventional treatments are available for prostate cancer?....Page 67

Expectant therapy...Page 68

Prostatectomy...Page 68

Radiation therapy...Page 69

External beam radiation...Page 69

Internal radiation therapy..Page 70

Hormone therapy...Page 70

Chemotherapy..Page 71

Safe and effective natural remedies can help you avoid
risky surgery..Page 72

Stem the growth of cancerous cells and reduce the size of
your prostate with these 4 incredible all-natural remedies...............Page 72

How a blend of the most powerful plant antioxidants – contained
in a tasty new drink – can help you fight prostate cancer...............Page 74

Healthy Cells Prostate™ helps maintain the health of your
prostate and reduces your risk of prostate cancer............................Page 77

Increase your intake of pomegranates to protect your prostate......Page 80

How a mushroom heralds an important breakthrough for
prostate cancer sufferers..Page 81

Discover the traditional Vietnamese medicine that may hold
the key to overcoming prostate and ovarian disorders...................Page 84

Wipe out prostate cancer without touching a single healthy cell?
An incredible new breakthrough looks set to do just that...............Page 87

Chapter Four: Breast Cancer......................................**Page 92**

Separating myth from fact to help protect you against the disease.......Page 92

Taking HRT could be increasing your risk of breast cancer
by up to 40%..Page 92

Exercise found to lower risk of premenopausal breast cancer........Page 94

Testing for breast cancer – what you need to know........................Page 95

Breast self-examination: An effective way to detect breast cancer?.....Page 95

Mammograms – an outdated and painful procedure......................Page 96

Genetics no longer thought to play a big role................................Page 98

Thermography: A safe and very effective alternative
to mammograms...Page 101

Breast Cancer Detection System (BCDS).....................................Page 104

What if an abnormality is found following screening?....................Page 105

What to expect if your doctor diagnoses breast cancer..................Page 105

How to combat anaemia caused by radiation therapy....................Page 107

Maximise your chances of beating breast cancer with
these natural remedies ....Page 109

Antioxidants may help guard against the disease ....Page 109

How protection from breast cancer could be found
from an unlikely source ....Page 110

Taking fish oil supplements can lower your risk of
breast cancer by up to 32% ....Page 111

Black cohosh can reduce your risk of breast cancer by over 60% ....Page 111

Vitamins and calcium supplements can lower breast cancer risk ..Page 112

Vitamin D helps block the growth of blood vessels that feed
breast cancer cells ....Page 112

Ginseng could improve breast cancer patients' quality of life ......Page 113

Indole-3-carbinol: A natural breakthrough in the fight
against breast cancer ....Page 115

Study shows how support groups improve the survival rates
of breast cancer patients ....Page 118

Breast-Mate™ – this ground-breaking mushroom remedy
helps stop breast cancer in its tracks ....Page 119

Two simple lifestyle changes that can help ward off breast cancer ..Page 123

Increase your chances of beating breast cancer with this
ground-breaking new complementary remedy ....Page 125

How a product derived from wheat germ is outperforming
many leading conventional drugs... including tamoxifen ....Page 128

New research shows pomegranate compounds kill breast
cancer cells – but beware, many pomegranate supplements
are a complete waste of money ....Page 132

Chapter Five: Skin Cancer ....Page 136

The lowdown on skin cancer... could your sunscreen be
doing you more harm than good? ....Page 136

The 3 main types of skin cancer and how to spot them ....Page 136

The sun produces your body's own defence against skin
cancer – vitamin D ....Page 137

New research questions the safety of many common ingredients found in sunscreens....................................Page 138

How to protect your skin during the summer months..............Page 139

VitaCell can protect your skin from sun-related damage – helping to lower your risk of skin cancer and wrinkles.................Page 140

Natural protection against sun damage – from the inside out!....Page 144

Chapter Six: Colon Cancer...**Page 148**

Colon cancer screening: new non-invasive method investigated....Page 149

What happens if you're diagnosed with colon cancer?...................Page 151

Colon cancer: Are you at risk? ....Page 152

How elevated levels of C-reactive protein could spell colon cancer..Page 152

Eating plenty of fibre can help ward off colon cancer.................Page 153

Men – lower your risk of colorectal cancer by eating more calcium and dairy...Page 155

Calcium may help prevent and treat polyps..............................Page 156

Animal studies indicate that dietary magnesium may protect against colon cancer...Page 157

These 5 key nutrients may prevent colorectal polyps from developing ....Page 158

4 simple ways to lower your risk of colon cancer.........................Page 159

Folic acid can help prevent cancerous colon polyps......................Page 161

Chapter Seven: Bladder Cancer ....**Page 163**

Causes of bladder cancer...Page 163

How is bladder cancer diagnosed...Page 164

Treating bladder cancer..Page 166

New research findings offer hope in the fight against bladder cancer..Page 168

Eat your way to a healthier bladder..Page 169

How cruciferous vegetables can lower your risk of bladder
cancer by up to 30%...Page 170

Chapter Eight: Cervical Cancer...................................Page 172

Cervical dysplasia: Don't panic if your smear test result shows
abnormalities... it doesn't necessarily spell cancer........................Page 172

The risk of cervical dysplasia developing into cancer is
extremely small..Page 172

The accuracy of your smear test can depend on where you live!......Page 173

Alternative approaches can help reverse cervical dysplasia and
lower your risk of cancer...Page 174

What to do if your smear test result shows an abnormality............Page 175

Gardasil® is not the 'fairytale cancer vaccine' it's dressed up to be..Page 176

Treatment options for cervical cancer...Page 178

Chapter Nine: Pancreatic Cancer – the 'silent disease'..Page 181

If pancreatic cancer is suspected, there are a number of tests
your doctor can carry out ....Page 181

The lowdown on the treatment options available..........................Page 182

Research uncovers simple ways to prevent pancreatic cancer.......Page 184

Enter vitamin D..Page 184

Another promising research finding in the fight against
pancreatic cancer..Page 185

Pancreatic cancer study update: How fish oil can reduce
symptoms of cachexia ....Page 186

Chapter Ten: Ovarian Cancer ....Page 188

Could you be at risk? ....Page 188

Diagnosing the disease ....Page 189

Ovarian cancer – treatment and recovery....................................Page 190

High folate intake can help ward off ovarian cancer.....................Page 191

Good news for tea lovers ....Page 193

Ovarian cancer protection from gingko....................Page 193

Get up and get moving..Page 194

Chapter Eleven: Lung Cancer.....................................Page 195

How to recognise the symptoms that can spell lung cancer........Page 196

How is lung cancer diagnosed?...................................Page 197

A new diagnostic tool identifies the earliest stages of lung
cancer with a non-invasive procedure........................Page 198

Four simple ways to keep your lungs disease-free.......................Page 199

Treatment options available.......................................Page 199

New hope for advanced lung cancer patients too sick
for chemotherapy..Page 200

How simple dietary changes can reduce your risk of lung cancer....Page 202

**Chapter Twelve: The natural anti-cancer therapies
showing real promise against the disease ....Page 204**

Vitamin C: A valuable addition to any anti-cancer arsenal...........Page 205

Should antioxidant supplements be avoided
during chemotherapy..Page 208

Antineoplaston therapy helps trigger the death of cancer cells....Page 210

Discover how your health could benefit from cutting-edge
enzyme therapy..Page 210

Ozone therapy delivers supercharged oxygen to your body...........Page 214

Gerson Therapy boosts the health of your liver and helps rid
your body of harmful toxins.......................................Page 217

Michael Gearin-Tosh's story of alternative cancer treatment.........Page 218

New research has revealed a link between low levels of
vitamin D and cancer...Page 221

Tocotrienols could reduce DNA damage that leads to cancer........Page 222

Essiac: Myth or Miracle?...Page 225

How a substance found in broccoli could revolutionise the
way we tackle cancer..Page 229

How the pulp and rind of citrus fruits have the ability to slow
or even halt the spread of cancer..Page 232

How a trace mineral is showing some truly 'miraculous'
results against cancer..Page 236

The plant that cancer researchers believe could hail a
breakthrough in the fight against the disease ....Page 239

Discover the latest research finding that led one leading
scientist to claim is: "The most significant breakthrough in
nutrition since the discovery of vitamins".....................................Page 242

How to take full advantage of pomegranate's anti-cancer and
anti-inflammatory properties..Page 245

Rhodiola rosea has a wide-range of health benefits and may
even protect against cancer..Page 249

Haelan 951 – a revolutionary new type of soya drink that
could offer vital protection against cancer....................................Page 251

Boost your immune system with "the most powerful
immune complex.. ever tested!"...Page 255

Discover how a weed is offering hope to countless
cancer sufferers...Page 258

How a little-known ingredient found in fruit and vegetables
can reduce your risk of cancer..Page 262

Ashwagandha: Exciting new research findings reveal how the
herb can help fight cancer..Page 265

A new supplement heralds good news for cancer and
diabetes sufferers..Page 267

How to safeguard your health from a diverse range of
diseases... including cancer...Page 270

This incredible Chinese mushroom could slash your risk
of cancer...Page 272

Another mushroom that is proving its worth in the fight
against cancer is Coriolus versicolor...Page 275

The natural remedy that could soon break into the mainstream
as a cancer treatment used alongside chemotherapy....................Page 278

Could this overlooked 'waste product' be the
cancer-fighting breakthrough of the century?.............................Page 282

How to overcome cancer-related fatigue..Page 286

Chinese plant may help fight cancer and ageing as well as
chronic diseases like arthritis and heart disease...........................Page 288

Perillyl alcohol – a natural compound found in cherries
may help fight cancer...Page 291

Discover the plant extract that is proving invaluable in
the fight against cancer...Page 294

Graviola: This Amazonian remedy provides potent
anti-cancer benefits...Page 296

Discover the superior form of cat's claw that defends against
disease by protecting and repairing your body's precious DNA...Page 300

**Chapter Thirteen: Much-needed relief from
cancer pain**..**Page 305**

Hypnotherapy – tap into the power of suggestion to
overcome discomfort..Page 306

Visualisation – picture yourself healthy, happy and pain free......Page 306

Herbal pain relief...Page 307

Herbal protection for chemo and radiation-therapy dangers..........Page 308

Zyflamend's remarkable pain-relieving and inflammation-
fighting properties can help cancer patients.................................Page 309

A final word of advice..**Page 314**

Further reading...**Page 316**

Helpful organisations..**Page 319**

Introduction

If you've been told you have cancer, or if someone in your family has, you're familiar with the emotional roller coaster you're suddenly thrown onto. It's a frightening prospect and can give rise to a whole range of strong emotions – shock, fear, anger, bitterness, confusion and depression.

These feelings are totally normal and can result from uncertainty about what the future holds and whether the cancer can be cured.

However, cancer shouldn't automatically be thought of as a death sentence… that's often far from being the case, especially if your cancer is caught early.

In fact, recent research findings by Cancer Research UK are extremely encouraging and indicate that real advances in effective cancer treatments are being made. Their research has indicated that survival rates for cancer patients have doubled in a generation, and that people with breast, bowel, or ovarian cancers are twice as likely to live for another 10 years than patients diagnosed in the 1970s were.

Taking all cancers together, almost half of patients diagnosed in 2007 can expect to live for 10 years after diagnosis compared with less than a quarter of those diagnosed in 1971-1972.

Maximise your chances of beating cancer

If you or a loved one has been diagnosed with cancer you need all the available information on the disease and the very best treatments for it at hand… it's not enough to simply cross your fingers, pray for a miracle and place your entire trust in the experts.

Knowledge really is power, especially when it comes to successfully fighting a disease like cancer, and can help you regain a sense of control. That's where *The Cancer Survival Manual – Tomorrow's Cancer Breakthroughs TODAY* can help.

You'll discover essential information and advice on the best conventional treatments available and the latest all-natural, complementary breakthroughs that are helping to win the war against the disease.

Complementary treatments are becoming increasingly popular, as many provide an effective way of boosting immunity. Your immune system is your body's first line of defence against cancer, as a strong immune system is better able to identify any cancerous cells and eliminate them before they have a chance to grow and spread. If you develop the disease all your body's resources, such as natural killer (NK) cells, are called upon to help fight the illness – in fact, a single NK cell can destroy up to 27 cancer cells before it dies. So it makes sense to strengthen your body's natural defences.

With individual chapters on specific types of cancer, you'll learn about new advances being made by both conventional and complementary medicine in each area... from the most accurate diagnostic testing procedures available, to the treatments that offer sufferers the best chance of making a successful recovery.

Rather than waste precious time trying to trawl through all the available research on the cancer preventatives and treatments out there that are making real inroads in the fight against the disease, we've done the hard work for you. With *The Cancer Survival Manual – Tomorrow's Cancer Breakthroughs TODAY* at your finger tips you'll have access to easy-to-follow, practical advice and potentially life-saving information.

Armed with this knowledge you can expect to feel empowered and confident that you can work alongside your doctor to make informed decisions about your health and about what care gives you the best chance of successfully fighting the disease. This is incredibly important as a positive mental attitude and a belief that you will get better has been found to play a key role in successful cancer healing outcomes.

We've also provided you with information on where to go to learn more, plus a list of helpful organizations and support groups. The latter can be particularly beneficial, as talking about your fears and concerns can go a long way to helping to reduce your anxiety. In addition, talking to others who have been in your situation can be useful as they will probably have a far greater understanding of how you feel and what you're going through than many of those closest to you. Better still, a US study revealed how breast cancer survivors had better survival rates when they participated in weekly talk group sessions with other cancer survivors and a clinical psychologist.

Discover simple measures that can keep you disease free

Even if you're not battling cancer then *The Cancer Survival Manual – Tomorrow's Cancer Breakthroughs TODAY* is an indispensible resource for remaining cancer free. This is extremely important, as according to Cancer Research UK one in three people are predicted to develop the disease at some stage in their life.

What makes this situation so tragic is that in many cases cancer is an entirely preventable disease simply by eating the right kind of foods, taking regular exercise and making healthy lifestyle choices... as you're about to find out.

Obviously, some risk factors like age and genetics are beyond your control, but cancer experts estimate that maintaining a healthy bodyweight, making dietary changes and taking regular physical activity could prevent about one in three deaths from cancer in the UK.

Avoiding known carcinogens is another important step. Risk factors linked to the disease include smoking, UV rays, pesticides, X-rays, living near power lines, fluoride in our drinking water, mobile phones, the contraceptive pill, medications like HRT and blood pressure drugs known as angiotensin receptor blockers *(Lancet 2003; 362: 419-427; Lancet 2005; 365: 1543-51; The Lancet Oncology, Early Online Publication, 14 June 2010)*, and chemicals in many cosmetics and household products – from lipstick to air fresheners.

In fact, according to the latest research findings published in the journal *Environmental Health*, women who regularly use a combination of certain cleaning products are twice as likely to develop breast cancer as women who rarely use these products. The US researchers found that the strongest link was between breast cancer and air fresheners and mould and mildew removers. Insect repellents, oven and surface cleaners also produced a slight increase.

While some of the other risk factors mentioned need more research to determine exactly how much of a threat they pose, it makes sense to take precautionary measures and minimize your exposure to them. So, in the case of mobile phones, make sure you don't carry yours around all day in your trouser pocket, where it is in such close proximity to your body, and opt for a hands-free device when making calls.

With *The Cancer Survival Manual – Tomorrow's Cancer Breakthroughs TODAY* you'll have access to all the latest cutting-edge research findings on how to prevent cancer, as well as what's been scientifically proven to be most successful at fighting established cases of the disease.

Chapter One: What is Cancer?

Cancer is a disease of the cells in your body. Your body contains millions of tiny cells, which each maintain their own existence and make vital contributions to your health. Healthy cells have a normal life cycle of approximately 120 days before they die. Your body then replaces these dying cells with healthy cells.

There are many different types of cells in your body, and there are many different types of cancer (around 200) which arise from different types of cells. What all types of cancer have in common is that the cancer cells are abnormal and grow at a quicker rate than healthy cells... multiplying 'out of control' and refusing to die.

A malignant tumour is a 'lump' or 'growth' of tissue made up from cancer cells which continue to divide and grow – making new blood vessels to feed themselves in a process called angiogenesis. Tumours that stay in one spot and demonstrate limited growth are generally considered to be benign.

Malignant tumours invade into nearby tissues which can cause damage and they can also spread to other parts of your body. This happens if some cells break off from the first 'primary' tumour and are carried in the bloodstream or lymph channels to other parts of your body. These small groups of cells may then multiply to form 'secondary' tumours (metastases) in one or more parts of your body. These secondary tumours may then grow, invade and damage nearby tissues, and spread again.

Cancer is not just one condition, and some forms of cancer are more serious than others, some are more responsive to treatment than others (particularly if diagnosed at an early stage), and some have a better outlook (prognosis) than others. In each case it is important to know exactly what type of cancer has developed, how large it has become, and whether it has spread to increase your chances of getting the most appropriate treatment and successfully beating it.

All in the genes?

Most types of cancer become more common as we get older. This is because the changes that make a cell become cancerous in the first place take a long time to develop.

There have to be a number of changes to the genes within a cell before it turns into a cancer cell. These changes can happen by accident when the cell is dividing. Or they can happen because the cell has been damaged by carcinogens and the damage is then passed on to future 'daughter' cells when that cell divides. The longer we live, the more time there is for genetic errors to occur in our cells.

However, bear in mind that cells often destroy themselves if they carry a mutation. Or the cells might be recognised by the immune system as abnormal and killed. This means most precancerous cells die before they can cause cancer. Only a small number of the changes turn into a cancer.

Sometimes a person is born with a genetic mutation within a cell. This doesn't mean they will definitely get cancer. But with one mutation from the start, it makes it more likely statistically that they will develop cancer during their lifetime. Doctors call this 'genetic predisposition'.

The BRCA1 and BRCA2 breast cancer genes are examples of genetic predisposition. Women who carry one of these faulty genes have a higher chance of developing breast cancer than women who do not.

The BRCA genes are good examples for another reason. Most women with breast cancer do not have a mutated BRCA1 or BRCA2 gene. Less than 5 per cent of all breast cancer is due to these genes. So although women with one of these genes are individually more likely to get breast cancer, most breast cancer is not caused by a high risk inherited gene fault.

This is true of other common cancers where some people have a genetic predisposition, such as colon cancer.

So what causes cells to multiply out of control and form a tumour?

Without a strong immune system – the cornerstone of good health – we are vulnerable to every passing bug and to mutations in the body which, if left unchecked, can lead to serious diseases like cancer.

We all have cancer cells in our body, but as German physician and cancer pioneer Dr Josef Issels claimed, a healthy body won't develop cancer because it has a defence system that can recognize cancer cells and reject them. Cancer can only develop in an unhealthy body or in one whose immune system is not functioning properly.

Your immune system is like a defending army, with resistance fighters based within both your bloodstream and your lymphatic system – a network of vessels which drains fluid back into your blood circulation.

The main defenders – white blood cells and lymphocytes – are constantly on the lookout for abnormal cells. White blood cells destroy micro-organisms by engulfing them. Lymphocytes can destroy foreign bodies directly or produce antibodies to inactivate undesirable substances, such as bacteria and viruses. Other cells, known as natural killer (NK) cells, directly attack and destroy cancer cells before they get the chance to multiply.

It's hardly surprising that cancer is the second biggest killer in the UK, when you realise that so much of modern living appears to be designed to weaken the immune system: air pollution, stress, smoking, the sun, radiation such as gamma and X-rays, compounds in car exhaust fumes, poor diet and environmental toxins can have a cumulative effect and cause a breakdown in immunity.

Scientists from the Harvard Medical School in Boston revealed, in a report published in the journal *Cancer Epidemiology, Biomarkers & Prevention*, that using talcum powder once a week raises the risk of womb cancer in older women by almost a quarter (24 per cent), as powder particles applied to the genital area can lead to inflammation, which allows cancer cells to grow.

When the body is exposed to carcinogens (cancer-causing substances) like these, damage occurs to the body's DNA. Free radicals are formed that try to steal electrons from other molecules in the body. These free radicals damage cells and affect their ability to function normally – instead of dying, the cells continue to divide and reproduce until they create a tumour.

However, what affects one body tissue may not affect another. For example, tobacco smoke that you breathe in may cause lung cancer, and overexposing your skin to the sun could cause a melanoma on your leg. But the sun won't give you lung cancer and smoking won't give you melanoma. Often there is more than one factor at work.

Just half an hour a day on your mobile could increase your risk of brain cancer by up to 40%

The debate about whether mobile phones can cause cancer is ongoing. However, the latest worrying research findings from the World Health Organization (WHO) warn of a direct link between cancer and heavy mobile phone use. The WHO commissioned scientists from around the globe to carry out a decade-long study. It involved more than 5,000 men and women with brain tumours from 13 different countries, as well as a similar number of healthy people, all of whom were interviewed about their phone habits.

The landmark report revealed that just half an hour a day on a mobile phone can increase a person's risk of brain cancer by up to 40 per cent. Those in the heaviest user category were in greater danger of developing malignant glioma tumours, which account for half of all brain tumours in the UK. The frequent users were also more likely to suffer a tumour on the same side of their brain to the ear they used for phone calls *(Published online, 17 May 2010, in the International Journal of Epidemiology).*

In the US, the Federal Communications Commission (FCC) acknowledges that cell (mobile) phones could present a serious health threat. They now recommend that people use an earpiece or headset with a mobile phone because "recent reports by some health and safety interest groups have suggested that wireless device use can be linked to cancer and other illnesses. These questions have become more pressing as more and younger people are using the devices and for longer periods".

The FCC's guidelines also advise users to keep phones away from the body: they should not attach them to a belt or leave them in a pocket that's next to the body. In addition, users are advised to use the speaker option so that the phone is held away from the head and, wherever possible, people should text rather than talk. The FCC also recommends that people purchase a phone with a lower SAR (specific absorption rate) *(www.fcc.gov/oet/rsafety/).*

Could the medical profession have got it wrong?

One unorthodox school of thought, which is becoming ever more popular in certain scientific circles (especially as more evidence emerges to back it up), is that bacteria may play a key role in the development of cancer and may even be a major cause of the disease

(Cancer Prev Res, 2008; 1:15-20, online; Mol Ther, 2010; April 13; doi: 10.1038/mt.2010.59).

Scientists that subscribe to this view believe that the disease is part of a process that begins when the body's own benign bacteria undergo a harmful cycle of transformation – triggered by known 'carcinogens' such as radiation, pollution and smoking – that progresses to inflammation and eventually cell mutation.

US researchers at the University of North Carolina believe that the 100 trillion bacterial organisms that normally reside benignly (mainly in the gut) can become hostile as a result of factors such as smoking or poor diet. They cite this as a major cause of colorectal cancer in particular *(Cancer Prev Res, 2008; 1 [7 supppl]: CN15-02; doi: 10.1158/1940-6207. PREV-08-CN15-02).*

If this theory is correct then it would radically change the way cancer is treated, with antibiotics replacing chemotherapy drugs as a first line treatment.

It is well established that some bacteria can cause certain cancers. For example, *Helicobacter pylori* bacteria can cause stomach cancer. Viruses also play a role – the hepatitis B virus is the culprit behind half of all liver cancers; and the human papillomavirus is a cause of cervical cancer.

However, Henry Pitot, a professor of oncology at the University of Wisconsin in the US, sums up the mainstream's overriding viewpoint on this issue when he says: "there is no evidence that bacteria, besides *H. pylori*, contribute to the development of cancer in any significant way" *(J Natl Cancer Inst, 2000; 92: 1713).*

Going back to the potential of antibiotics to treat cancer... a study has already proven that antibiotics can play an integral part in the treatment process of gastric cancer caused by the *Helicobacter pylori* bacteria.

In a study of 544 patients who had undergone stomach-cancer surgery, antibiotics reduced the risk of a second cancer by two-thirds. Half of the patients were given a course of the antibiotics lansoprazole, amoxicillin and clarithromycin; while the remaining half received standard care but no drug treatment for *H. pylori*. Three years later, cancer had recurred in nine patients in the group administered antibiotics, compared with 24 patients in the standard care group *(Lancet, 2008; 372: 392-7)*.

What about other forms of cancer? In 2009, US researchers at the Johns Hopkins University in Baltimore found that a species of bacteria called *Bacteroides fragilis*, which commonly inhabits the human intestinal tract, can cause colon cancer. Commenting on the findings, lead researcher Cynthia Sears, said: "This could be the *H. pylori* of colon cancer". In an animal study, the bacteria was found to cause chronic inflammation, which in turn damages genetic material in the colon cells, allowing them to grow uncontrollably and to develop into tumours. The bacteria have been found in the gut of up to 35 per cent of children and adults, and 40 per cent of colon cancer patients *(Nat med, 2009; 15: 1016-22)*.

The theory that bacteria may be behind many types of cancer continues to be largely ignored by mainstream medicine, despite the fact that it has very few answers of its own when it comes to cancer.

Mainstream medicine's approach to fighting the disease

Cancer treatment has come a long way since the use of mustard gas derivatives in the early 1900s – or has it? Despite all the drugs, research and money invested in finding a cure for cancer, the search for the magic bullet has so far proved futile.

When doctors discovered during World War One that mustard gas destroyed bone marrow, they began to experiment with it as a way to kill cancer cells. Although they had little success with the mustard gas, it did pave the way for modern chemotherapy – which involves the most toxic and poisonous substances anyone deliberately puts in their body.

While these toxic chemicals are able to zap cancer cells they also have a devastating effect on healthy cells. The side effects of these chemicals vary according to the drug given, but they can, ironically, further suppress the immune system (a process known as immunosuppression).

Chemotherapy is often used in conjunction with radiation treatment, which targets cancer cells using X-rays or gamma rays to deter the proliferation of malignant cells. It is not unusual to experience common side effects from this treatment, including nausea, vomiting and hair loss.

Medicinal drugs may also be prescribed, which can be harsh on the body and add to the toxic load.

Surgery is another treatment option that involves removing the tumour and surrounding tissue.

In some cases cancer can come back after treatment. It may come back in the same area in which it first started, this is known as a recurrence. This can happen because tiny cancer cells, that may have been left behind when the tumour was removed, or that weren't destroyed by treatments such as radiotherapy and chemotherapy, have begun to divide again and form a tumour.

Some types of cancer grow very slowly and may cause no problems for many years. In this situation you may not need to have any treatment for some time, but your doctor will monitor you closely so that if the cancer does start to grow you can be given treatment at that time.

Chapter Two: Diet

The disease-fighting nutrients that provide a vital defence against cancer

The importance of diet when it comes to cancer prevention can't be emphasized enough. It should also play a key role in fighting established cases of the disease.

The World Health Organisation (WHO) has revealed that 85 per cent of adult cancers are entirely avoidable and, of these, around half are related to nutritional deficiencies in the Western diet.

By contrast, an impressive body of research has revealed that those people who eat the recommended serving of five fruits and vegetables a day (as a minimum) are half as likely to develop cancer as those who eat the least amount of these foods.

Healthy eating tips – your way to 5 a day

- It can sometimes be difficult to squeeze in all five portions. But fresh, frozen, chilled, canned, 100 per cent juice and smoothies all count, as do dried fruit and veg. Although bear in mind that potatoes don't count at all. Plus pasta sauces and fresh and tinned soups also contribute to your five a day – but check the nutritional information on the labels as you don't want to undo the goodness with lots of sugar, fat or salt. Around 80g of fruit and veg in a product counts as a portion.

- A portion of vegetables is three heaped tablespoons of carrots, peas or sweetcorn, or a cereal bowl of mixed salad. Three heaped tablespoons of beans and pulses such as lentils and chick peas also count as a portion, but only count them once a day, even if you eat all three. That's because pulses don't contain as many nutrients.

- A portion of fruit is one medium apple or banana, two small satsumas or three dried apricots. You can only count a glass of 100 per cent fruit juice once a day, however many flavours you drink. Fibre is removed in processing so it's not as nutritious as a piece of fruit. A portion of dried fruit is one tablespoon but stick to one a day as it is high in sugar.

- Try something new every week. There are bound to be lots of fruit and veg varieties that you've never tasted – so vary what you buy and eat, rather than get into a rut of buying the same five things every time you go to the greengrocers. Aim for as many colours and textures as possible and five different choices every day. For example, five bananas would still only count as one portion.

- It's also important to point out that the way you cook your veggies is vital in order to unlock their full goodness. Make sure you steam your vegetables rather than boil them, otherwise you risk losing many of the important nutrients they contain. If you do boil vegetables, the cooking water should be used for another culinary purpose, since boiling causes the leaching of the minerals they contain into the cooking water. For example, use the water for soup making. Stir frying is OK as long as you do not cook over a very high temperature and only cook the vegetables for a few minutes.

- Serving your vegetables raw may offer the best way to help you take full advantage of their anti-cancer properties. The plant-based medicines in vegetables are delicate molecules that are easily destroyed by heat. For example, microwaving broccoli destroys up to 98 per cent of its phytonutrients (components that promote health), including its anti-cancer nutrients. US researchers from the Roswell Park Cancer Institute in Buffalo discovered that eating raw cruciferous vegetables can decrease the risk of developing bladder cancer by 40 per cent. The researchers conducted a survey on the eating habits of 1,100 people, 275 of whom had bladder cancer. They found that among both smokers and non-smokers, those who ate three or more servings of raw cruciferous vegetables each month had a 40 per cent lower risk of developing bladder cancer. Compared with smokers who did not eat that amount, non-smokers who ate three or more servings of raw cruciferous vegetables per month had a 73 per cent lower chance of developing bladder cancer. These cruciferous anti-cancer nutrients only stay in the body for about 12 hours, which indicates that the participants only experienced a total of about 36 hours with these nutrients (out of a total of 720 hours in a typical month). In other words, they only had these anti-cancer nutrients in their bodies 5 per cent of the time. Astonishingly their bladder cancer rates plummeted by 40 per cent and keep in mind that the research only involved three servings of raw cruciferous vegetables a month. Remarkably, the researchers did not find a protective benefit from eating the same quantity of cooked cruciferous vegetables. This indicates that the anti-cancer properties of cruciferous vegetables may be destroyed during the cooking process.

What you don't eat is just as important as what you do eat

The latest research findings have revealed that consuming too many processed meats can increase the risk of bowel and pancreatic cancer. In fact, eating just one sausage a day increases your risk of bowel cancer by up to 20 per cent.

Many people are leaving themselves incredibly vulnerable to obesity, cancer and a lifetime of ill-health as a result of their heavy reliance on junk food and chemically-treated, processed foods. As well as having little (if any) nutritional value they're typically laden with too much fat, refined sugar and salt, not to mention all the artificial colourings, flavourings and preservatives.

This leaves your poor body overwhelmed with the task of getting rid of all these harmful toxins, which places a huge burden on important organs like your liver and kidneys. As a result your body has less time to get on with its usual important tasks of cleansing, healing and renewal.

Obviously one of the best ways to achieve peak health and prevent cancer is to take regular exercise and follow a varied and balanced diet, which includes plenty of fresh, wholefoods – choosing organic and seasonal foods whenever possible. It should be rich in whole grains, nuts, seeds, fruits and vegetables which are high in antioxidants – natural chemicals that bolster your immune system and help fight harmful 'cancer-causing' free radicals.

The anti-cancer rainbow diet

A cancer-protective diet should also contain different coloured fruits and vegetables, which provide a broad spectrum of essential nutrients.

For example, fruit and veg that are yellow/orange in colour – like peaches, apricots, nectarines, pineapples, mangoes, oranges, carrots, butternut squash, sweet potatoes and peppers – contain high amounts of cancer-fighting antioxidants including vitamin C, carotenoids and bioflavonoids.

Foods high in these nutrients help bolster your body's defences and, according to the World Cancer Research Fund and American Institute for Cancer Research (AICR), they help reduce the risk of various gut and lung cancers.

Fruit and veg with a blue/purple-black colour, such as plums, blueberries, blackberries, raisins, prunes and aubergines contain health-promoting phytochemicals (natural plant compounds) such as anthocyanins and phenolics, which have disease-fighting and anti-ageing benefits.

And red-rich tomatoes and watermelon are important providers of lycopene – a pigment in plants that helps reduce the risk of prostate cancer, according to a report by the World Cancer Research Fund.

According to Karen Collins, MS, RD, nutritional advisor to the

AICR: "Vegetables and fruits, along with whole grains, beans, nuts and seeds, contain thousands of phytochemicals – many of which influence one or more stages of cancer development. This makes variety in the plant foods we eat more important than ever."

The AICR recommends meals in which two-thirds of your plate is made up of fruits, vegetables, whole grains and beans. The following list shows those foods that are particularly beneficial in terms of their cancer-fighting properties:

Allicin
Found In: Garlic, leek, onion, scallion, shallot
Actions: Garlic intake linked to reduced cancer rates; allyl sulfides suppress wild cell growth

---

A pungent reminder: garlic remains a potent player in the fight against cancer

Garlic has long been known for its ability to stimulate the immune system. Research is under way to investigate garlic (*allium sativum*) for the treatment of bladder cancer (*Urol Clin North Am, Feb. 2000*).

According to the sponsoring doctors at the Department of Urology, Robert C. Byrd Health Science Center, the list of garlic's beneficial effects include detoxification of chemical carcinogens, prevention of carcinogenesis, inhibition of cancer cell growth, protection against tumour growth, and protection against the damaging effects of radiation therapy and chemotherapy. A powerful agent indeed, and one worth continued attention for its ever-broadening health applications.

Limonoids
Found In: Grapefruit, lemon, lime, noni, orange
Actions: Promotes detoxification of cancer-causing compounds within the digestive tract; may inhibit breast cancer cell growth

How the health benefits of oranges
extend beyond vitamin C

Oranges are one of Mother Nature's best super foods, packed with an unbelievable array of disease-fighting nutrients, all tucked neatly beneath the peel. The fruit has long been known to be a rich source of immune-boosting vitamin C, which plays an important role in cancer prevention.

Now, Californian scientists have discovered that oranges are also rich in compounds called citrus limonoids. These chemicals have been proven to help fight a number of varieties of cancer, including that of the mouth, skin, lung, breast, stomach and colon.

The researchers have found that each time we bite into a citrus slice or drink a glass of orange juice, our bodies can readily access a limonoid called limonin, which as well as having cancer-fighting properties can also help lower cholesterol.

Carotenoids
Found In: Apricots, carrots, kale, spinach, sweet potatoes
Actions: Antioxidants that boost immunity; one carotenoid, lutein, has been linked to reduced risk of kidney and ovarian cancers

How eating more spinach could reduce
ovarian cancer risk

Spinach is one of the most nutritious of the leafy green vegetables – it's packed full of calcium, folic acid, vitamin K, energy-promoting iron, vitamin C, fibre, carotenoids, lutein and bioflavonoids.

The A and C vitamins in spinach plus the fibre, folic acid, magnesium and other nutrients help control cancer, especially colon, lung and breast cancers.

Spinach's secret weapon, a carotenoid called lutein, makes it one of the best foods to prevent cataracts, as well as age-related macular degeneration, the leading cause of preventable blindness in the elderly. As already mentioned, foods rich in lutein also appear to help protect against cancer, including kidney and ovarian cancers.

Now the latest research findings have revealed that an increased intake of the flavonoid kaempferol, which is found in spinach, is associated with a 40 per cent reduced risk of ovarian cancer.

Ovarian cancer accounts for 4 per cent of all cancers diagnosed in women globally, with 190,000 new cases every year. In Europe there are 61,000 new cases each year, with the highest incidence rates found in the Northern European countries of the UK, Ireland, Denmark and Finland.

The new study, led by Margaret Gates from Brigham and Women's Hospital and Harvard Medical School, fills a gap in our knowledge since no prospective study has previously examined the association between flavonoid intake and ovarian cancer risk.

Gates and co-workers calculated intake of the flavonoids myricetin, kaempferol, quercetin, luteolin and apigenin among 66,940 women enrolled in the Nurses' Health Study. Between 1984 and 2002, 347 cases of epithelial ovarian cancer were diagnosed.

While total intake of the five flavonoids together was not found to provide a benefit, a significant 40 per cent reduction in ovarian cancer incidence was observed between the women with the highest kaempferol intake, compared to women with the lowest intake.

A significant 34 per cent reduction in ovarian cancer incidence was also observed between the women with the highest intake of the flavone luteolin (found in citrus, for example), compared to women with the lowest intake.

Commenting on the findings, Gates said: "There was evidence of an inverse association with consumption of tea (non-herbal) and broccoli, the primary contributors to kaempferol intake in our population. These data suggest that dietary intake of certain flavonoids may reduce ovarian cancer risk, although additional prospective studies are needed to further evaluate this association. If confirmed, these results would provide an important target for ovarian cancer prevention."

For optimal nutrition eat spinach raw – such as in sandwiches (in place of lettuce), or in salads. For a delicious spinach salad, toss baby spinach leaves with avocado, pistachio nuts and shaved parmesan cheese. You can always add some olives or sun-dried tomatoes for extra flavour.

Please note: People with kidney or bladder stones should avoid spinach because its oxalic content can exacerbate stones.

Catechins
Found In: Apples, berries, green tea
Actions: Inhibits enzymatic reactions that can lead to cancer; has
    reduced tumour size in laboratory studies

Green tea helps destroy breast cancer and oesophageal cancer cells

Green tea contains anti-cancer polyphenols, the most important of which is called epigallocatechin gallate (EGCG). Recent studies have found that green tea extract effectively destroys breast cancer cells in the laboratory (*J Agric Food Chem. 2007; 55(2): 243-253*) and reduces the size of breast cancer tumours in mice (*J Agric Food Chem.*

2007; 55(9): 3378-3385).

An epidemiological study in South-East China, concluded that the regular consumption of green tea has a protective effect against breast cancer *(Carcinogenesis 2007; 28(5): 1074-1078).*

Research has revealed another type of cancer that green tea can help fight – oesophageal cancer. The oesophagus is the muscular tube that propels food from your mouth to your stomach. In particular, the researchers found that green tea is able to inhibit oesophageal cancer associated with a condition called Barrett's oesophagus – chronic irritation of the oesophagus caused by heartburn and acid reflux.

Dr Howard Y Chang and colleagues who conducted the study at the Harvard Medical School and the Veterans Administration Boston Healthcare System in the US, believe that the oesophagus may benefit from being exposed to the high levels of polyphenols, such as EGCG, in green tea. EGCG in particular, is believed to block the production of an enzyme needed for cancer cells to grow. It is also thought to suppress the production of blood vessels that supply blood to cancer cells.

The scientists administered varying concentrations of EGCG to human Barrett's oesophagus-associated adenocarcinoma (cancerous) cells in the laboratory, and compared them to untreated cells. They found that cell growth was inhibited within 72 hours after exposure to EGCG. The team concluded that EGCG also induced cell death, which occurred as early as 24 hours after the treated cells were exposed to the compound.

Commenting on the results, Dr Chang said: "Research suggests that drinking green tea may be both a valuable chemopreventive therapy as well as a treatment for oesophageal adenocarcinoma. Our results suggest that extracts in green tea may help to lower the prevalence of oesophageal adenocarcinoma, one of the fastest growing cancers in

Western countries."

Drink three cups of green tea a day, or take 400mg to 800mg of standardised green tea extract daily.

Chlorophyll
Found In: Barley and wheat grasses, chlorella, leafy greens, spirulina
Actions: Helps neutralize toxins and boosts the body's immune defences

Eat your dark leafy greens to ward off prostate cancer

As well as toxin-fighting chlorophyll, dark leafy green vegetables are also a rich source of folate.

Folate is the form of the B vitamin folic acid that naturally occurs in foods, like spinach. Folic acid is essential for the proper synthesis and repair of DNA and therefore for cell division.

New findings published recently, report that there is a link between consuming a greater amount of folate with a reduced risk of developing prostate cancer.

A team of Italian researchers analysed data from 1,294 patients with diagnosed prostate cancer in comparison to 1,451 patients with growths (but not associated with tumours or cancer) who were admitted to the same hospital, in a case-control study of prostate cancer over a period of 11 years.

Researchers then evaluated over 78 different foods that had been eaten by these patients up to two years prior to their diagnosis or hospital admission. Folate intake was found to be directly related to prostate cancer risk. Researchers found that men who included a lot of folate in their diets had a 34 per cent lower risk of prostate cancer, compared to men whose intake of folate was considerably lower.

Based on these findings the researchers concluded that there is indeed a strong relationship between a high intake of folate and lower levels of cancer.

Firstly, the study concluded that a deficiency of folic acid decreases S-adenosylmethionine (SAMe), which can increase the level of activation of the genes that promote cancer. The other benefit from eating more folate is that a deficiency can trigger an error in DNA synthesis that leads to breaks in the chromosomes, which in turn can lead to an increase in developing prostate cancer.

In supplement form the recommended dose for folic acid is 400mcg daily, preferably taken at mealtimes.

Sulforaphane
Found In: Broccoli, especially broccoli sprouts
Actions: Has counteracted genes that increase cancer susceptibility in lab studies; helps the body destroy abnormal cells

How a substance found in broccoli can slow the spread of breast cancer by up to 90%!

Broccoli is a rich source of sulforaphane, which is thought to help prevent cancer by boosting the production of phase 2 enzymes within cells, which detoxify carcinogens and free radicals.

Broccoli's cancer-fighting benefits don't end there...

Postmenopausal women who eat brassica vegetables (such as broccoli, cabbage, cauliflower or Brussels sprouts) every day reduce their risk of breast cancer by up to 40 per cent, according to recent research at the Karolinska Institute in Stockholm, Sweden (*JAMA 285: 2975-7, 2001*).

Brassica vegetables are high in a compound called indole-3-carbinol (I3C) which stimulates the conversion of oestrone, the 'bad' form of oestrogen that promotes breast cancer, into an inactive form called 2-hydroxyoestrone *(Breakspear Medical Bulletin, Summer 2002).*

When researchers injected three groups of breast cancer cells with the drug tamoxifen, or I3C, or a combination of both, they saw cell growth inhibited by 60 per cent with tamoxifen, 90 per cent with I3C and 95 per cent with the combination *(Cancer Res. 59: 1244-51, 1999).* This suggests that I3C, which is available as a supplement, may be a better option than tamoxifen as a preventive treatment for women at high risk of breast cancer. Take 250mg a day.

Brassica vegetables also contain another anti-cancer substance called calcium D-glucarate. One of the ways that your body removes excess oestrogen is by bonding it to glucuronic acid in your liver and excreting it in your bile. However, as the resulting complex passes through your gut, an enzyme (beta-glucuronidase) produced by the resident bacteria breaks the bond and releases the oestrogen again.

Calcium D-glucarate inhibits that enzyme, so allowing excess oestrogen to be removed efficiently. Tests on animals have found that supplements of calcium D-glucarate can prevent the development of experimentally-induced cancers *(Cancer Lett. 49: 51-7, 1990).* Take 200-400mg a day as a preventive dose.

For more information on broccoli's cancer-fighting properties, see pages 115, 127 and 229.

Lycopene
Found In: Grapefruit, tomato, watermelon
Actions: Helps protect cells against free-radical damage; may reduce risk of breast, intestinal, pancreatic and prostate cancers

Why tomatoes could protect you from prostate cancer

Lycopene, the pigment that causes the red colour in tomatoes, plays a major role in maintaining the health of the prostate gland. A past study suggests that lycopene supplements could reduce the growth of prostate cancer. Patients scheduled for prostate removal received a 15mg lycopene supplement twice a day for three weeks. They experienced an average 20 per cent drop in their PSA levels and their tumours began to shrink *(Cancer Epidemiol Biomarkers Prev 2001; 10: 861-8)*.

Make tomatoes a regular part of your diet, preferably cooked and with added olive oil in order to increase the amount of lycopene you absorb. Alternatively, you can take a supplement of 30mg a day.

Ellagic acid
Found In: Grapes, pomegranates, raspberries, strawberries
Actions: Inhibits tumour growth and blood-vessel development, and promotes natural death of cancer cells, in laboratory studies

Ellagic acid heralds a vital breakthrough in the prevention of cancer

After years of intensive research, scientists have reported that ellagic acid – a natural compound found in high amounts in the leaves and seeds of raspberries, strawberries, pomegranates and other plant foods – is a powerful antioxidant that is able to bind to cancer-causing chemicals and neutralise them, thereby rendering them harmless *(Cancer Res. 2001; 61(16): 6112-6119)*.

In an animal study, American researchers from the College of Pharmacy, University of Toledo, Ohio, discovered that ellagic acid together with another potent antioxidant, vitamin E, is able to protect against a rather ominous-sounding cancer-causing chemical called 'tetrachlorodibenzo-dioxin' (*J Toxicol Environ Health A. 2006; 69(5): 381-93*).

Cancer is an extremely complex disease and there are literally thousands of different chemicals, including tetrachlorodibenzo-dioxin, involved in its development. Another one is casein kinase 2 (CK2). This is found in many tissues in your body and ordinarily doesn't pose a threat. It is only if it becomes activated that it increases your chances of cancer developing. The good news is that ellagic acid has been found to completely block the action of CK2 – even when it has already been activated (*Med Chem. 2006 Apr 20; 49(8): 2363-6*).

Encourages the death of cancerous cells while leaving healthy cells intact

Another way ellagic acid helps ward off cancer is by encouraging a natural process called apoptosis (natural cell death). Studies have found that ellagic acid forces cancerous cells to go through the normal apoptosis process without damaging healthy cells (*J Agric Food Chem. 2006; 54(3): 980-5*).

This is in contrast to many conventional cancer treatments, including chemotherapy, which cause the death of cancer cells and healthy cells indiscriminately, which can have a detrimental effect on the immune system.

The recommended dosage for ellagic acid (derived from concentrated red raspberry seed extract) is 1g tablet taken four times a day. This provides the equivalent of one cupful of fresh red raspberries a day (40mg of pure ellagic acid).

Resveratrol
Found In: Grapes and peanuts
Actions: Helps reduce exposure to the toxic effects of cancer-causing
chemicals and normalizes the natural cell life cycle

Resveratrol showing promise in the fight against breast, bowel and liver cancers

Recent research shows that resveratrol may be a useful plant chemical to use against several types of cancer. Resveratrol is thought to work in a variety of ways to reduce the likelihood of cancer.

For example, it can help block the supply of blood to the cancerous growth, thereby causing any cancer to wither and die. It also, for some unknown reason, attacks and destroys cancerous cells while at the same time allowing normal healthy cells to remain unharmed.

In a study published by researchers from the Faculty of Health Sciences, University Hospital, Linkoping in Sweden, the scientists observed a significantly lower breast cancer growth in cells treated with resveratrol. The scientists concluded that their study "supports the potential use of resveratrol as a chemotherapeutic agent in breast cancer" *(Cancer Lett 2006; 231(1): 113-22)*.

Other scientists have found that resveratrol works in different stages of bowel cancer and blocks several steps in the development of that cancer *(Sengottuvelan M, et al. Carcinogenesis, published online 7 December 2005)*.

French researchers from the University Victor Segalen in Bordeaux reported that resveratrol is also active against liver cancer in humans *(Int J Biochem Cell Biol 2006; 38(4): 629-37)*. They believe that resveratrol blocks the chemical signals between cancerous cells. This confuses their growth patterns and does not allow them to multiply.

Finally, certain scientists believe that resveratrol works by making cancer cells more sensitive to conventional chemotherapy drugs *(Antioxid Redox Signal 2005; 7(11-12): 1630-47)*.

So how much resveratrol do you need to receive these protective benefits? A glass of red wine provides about 640mcg but resveratrol supplements are available too if you prefer not to get your RDA from an alcoholic source. The recommended dose is 200mcg-600mcg daily.

Anthocyanins

Found In: Açai, berries, blackcurrants, goji, grapes, mangosteen, plums
Actions: May inhibit tumorous cell growth and protect against the kind of genetic damage that leads to cancer development

The secret of blueberry's 4-pronged attack on cancer

Most antioxidants can influence cancer growth and the ingredients in blueberries are particularly effective in stopping cancer growth on several fronts *(J Food Sci 2000, 65: 352-356)*:

- They discourage cancer cells from appearing in the first place, through a mechanism as yet to be fully researched.

- They shield healthy cells against injury by deactivating the free radicals produced by abnormal, cancerous cells.

- They block the formation of new blood vessels, which are needed by the fast-growing cancer cells, and so starve these cells of nutrients.

- They boost the immune system, which, in turn, attacks existing cancer cells and eliminates them.

Why all good things come to those who wait...

While just about every piece of health advice you read recommends lots of fresh fruits and vegetables, if you really want to get the most nutritional value out of them, you might want to adjust your definition of 'fresh'.

According to a study published in the *Journal of Agricultural and Food Chemistry*, some fruits and vegetables actually get better for you after they've been stored for a while. Not long enough for them to spoil, of course, but the researchers found that when they stored produce either at room temperature or in the refrigerator for several days, not only did the antioxidant capacity not go down (as anticipated), but some of the produce's flavonoid content actually increased.

Flavonoids are compounds in fruits and vegetables that give them their colour. They also have antioxidant properties. Which means that storing your fruits and vegetables for a few days before you eat them could be a simple way to boost your antioxidant intake – and, in turn, help ward off all the problems that come along with the free radical damage those antioxidants fight: conditions like cancer.

And if this research looks promising for 'regular' fruits and vegetables, imagine how a few days' storage could affect organic produce, which already has a nutritional leg-up on commercially grown varieties thanks to an absence of pesticides and herbicides.

Why opting for organic produce is worth the extra pennies

There are many health advantages to buying organic foods, plus it has never been easier now that there is an increased availability of fresh organic produce. More and more agricultural land is being turned over to organic production and more and more supermarket chains now stock a large range of organic produce.

Organic farming methods mean that crops are not subjected to pesticides, insecticides, fungicides and herbicides – all of which have been linked to cancer.

In addition to reducing the risk of toxicity, organic meat is a good way of ensuring that you are not consuming animals that have been given antibiotics to promote growth. As well as having negative effects on health, these antibiotics increase the resistant strains of bacteria that are now rapidly appearing. It also means no hormones or other medicinal drugs will be present in the meat. Plus, from an animal welfare point of view, organic farming methods mean that animals are treated in a more natural and humane way.

Organic produce also ensures fertilizers aren't being used, which deplete the soil of vital nutrients like selenium, zinc, magnesium and chromium. Currently in the UK organic foods also have to be free from genetically modified produce. Although the full potential risks from genetically modified foods have yet to be unveiled by research, there is a possibility that they may contain substances toxic to humans.

All genuinely organic food in the UK will be labelled as such and should carry the Soil Association symbol to show that it has been certified as organic. You may also see the term 'conservation grade' labelled on food products. This means the same as the organic label but shows that the farming practices used also employ additional measures to conserve the surrounding environment.

If you see the term 'transitional' labelled on a food item then this means that the food has come from a place where organic practices are being used but that it has not yet completed the full two-year changeover period. To be certified as organic there are strict regulations and guidelines that must be followed, and there is a two-year conversion period when these principles are applied but the product cannot be labelled as organic until this deadline has been reached.

While most of us choose organic foods usually because of what ISN'T in them – pesticides, growth hormones, and antibiotics, just to name a few choice harmful chemicals – new research suggests that we might get even more benefit from organically-grown fruits and vegetables because of what IS in them… a substance that might help protect us from cancer.

In a recent issue of the *British Journal of Nutrition*, researchers reported on their assessment of 35 different brands of vegetable soup, both organic and non-organic. They found that on average, the organic brands contained nearly six times as much salicylic acid, a natural anti-inflammatory agent.

The 11 organic brands tested boasted an average of 117 nanograms per gram of salicylic acid, while the 24 non-organic brands only contained an average of 20 ng/g. One soup in particular contained nearly 50 times the concentration of salicylic acid as in the average non-organic soup; the carrot and coriander soup from Scotland's Simply Organic contained 1,040 ng/g.

Previous research has shown that salicylic acid can help fight certain types of cancer. More and more studies are suggesting that the body's inflammatory response plays a critical role in many types of chronic disease. And earlier work by the same British research team proved that eating salicylic-rich foods translates into higher blood concentrations of the acid, so there is substantial reason to add this new finding to organic produce's list of benefits.

The researchers theorise that organic fruits and vegetables contain more salicylic acid because plants produce the substance as a natural defence mechanism. Without pesticides and other chemicals to keep insects and disease at bay, organically grown plants must protect themselves in order to thrive. This may explain why these plants contain so much more of this beneficial acid.

This study shows that what Mother Nature puts INTO our foods is just as important as what she doesn't. And if you've been unsure whether there was enough benefit to pay the additional cost of organic, here's another reason to consider it. Many supermarket chains across the country now offer organic produce right next to the conventionally grown fruits and vegetables. In most cases, you don't have to go out of your way to eat organic anymore – but even if you do, this research shows us that the benefits are even greater than we thought.

New research findings suggest that reducing your calorie intake by just 5% could lower your risk of cancer

The latest research findings offer fresh hope in the fight against cancer. US researchers from the University of California, Berkeley, found that reducing the number of calories in the diets of mice by just 5 per cent was almost as effective as reducing overall calorie intake by a third in preventing cell proliferation – an indicator of cancer risk.

Lead investigator and professor of nutrition Marc Hellerstein, of the Department of Nutritional Sciences and Toxicology at UC Berkeley's College of Natural Resources explained: "Cell proliferation is really the key to the modern epidemic of cancer. Normally, a cell will try to fix any damage that has occurred to its DNA. But if it divides before it has a chance to fix the damage, then that damage becomes memorialised as a mutation in the offspring cells [this is what is known as cell proliferation]. Slowing down the rate of cell proliferation essentially buys time for the cells to repair genetic damage."

In past animal studies, reducing total calorie intake by up to 50 per cent has been found to reduce the risk of cell proliferation and cancer, as well as lengthen lifespan. The current research suggests that these benefits could be achieved without having to severely restrict the total amount of calories consumed.

The US researchers fed one group of mice intermittently, which provided them with 5 per cent fewer calories than those consumed by another group of mice that were allowed to eat as much as they desired. A third group of mice were fed diets containing 33 per cent fewer calories than those consumed by the latter.

The researchers found that consuming 5 per cent fewer calories was nearly as effective as the more stringent 33 per cent calorie restriction in reducing cell proliferation in breast, skin and T-cells (immune cells derived from the thymus gland), compared to the mice that could eat as much as they liked.

Commenting on the findings, lead author Elaine Hsieh says, "cutting just a few calories overall but feeding intermittently may be a more feasible eating pattern for some people to maintain." *(American Journal of Physiology-Endocrinology and Metabolism, May 2005.)*

More anti-cancer foods to add to your shopping list...

- **Study findings uncover cancer-fighting properties linked to avocados**

Avocados are considered by many to be an almost complete food. This is hardly surprising given that they are a rich source of vitamins, minerals and phytonutrients, providing 4 per cent of the recommended Daily Value (DV) for vitamin E, 4 per cent vitamin C, 8 per cent folate, 4 per cent fibre, 2 per cent iron, 4 per cent potassium, with 81mcg of lutein and 19mcg of beta-carotene. They are renowned for their cholesterol-lowering properties and ability to maintain cardiovascular health.

According to the latest research findings from Dr Steven M. D'Ambrosio and his associates at Ohio State University, in the US, it appears that phytochemicals extracted from the popular Haas avocado are able to destroy oral cancer cells as well as prevent precancerous cells from developing into cancer *(report published online ahead of print in the journal Seminars in Cancer Biology)*.

Hass avocados are year-round fruits known for their distinctive bumpy skin that turns from green to purplish-black as they ripen. While there are more than 500 varieties of avocados grown worldwide, Hass avocados are the most readily available at supermarkets nationwide. Similar research has not been conducted on other varieties of avocados as yet, so it is not clear if these benefits are limited to Hass avocados alone or extend to all types.

For the purpose of this study, Dr D'Ambrosio, who is a member of the molecular carcinogenesis and chemoprevention program at OSU's Comprehensive Cancer Center, collaborated with Haiming Ding of the Department of Radiology, Young-Won Chin of the College of Pharmacy, and A. Douglas Kinghorn, also of the Comprehensive Cancer Center. They determined that the avocado compounds target multiple signalling pathways and increase intracellular reactive oxygen in precancerous cells to trigger programmed cell death, while leaving healthy cells unharmed.

Commenting on the findings, Dr D'Ambrosio said: "As far as we know, this is the first study of avocados and oral cancer. We think these phytochemicals either stop the growth of precancerous cells in the body or they kill the precancerous cells without affecting normal cells. Our study focuses on oral cancer, but the findings might have implications for other types of cancer. These are preliminary findings, and more research is needed."

- **Researchers reveal how watercress plays a vital role in the prevention of cancer**

Gram for gram, watercress contains as much vitamin C as oranges, more calcium than milk and more iron than spinach. It's a good source of folic acid, and is literally bursting with beta-carotene and vitamin A equivalents, which help promote healthy skin and eyes. It also contains antioxidants, which can help to mop up potentially harmful free radicals, and compounds known as glucosinolates which appear to have anti-cancer properties.

Researchers from the University of Ulster, in Northern Ireland, recently discovered that consuming watercress on a regular basis can prevent DNA damage – a key risk factor in the development of cancer *(American Journal of Clinical Nutrition, Feb 2007, Vol 85, No 2, Pages 504-510).*

The study involved 30 healthy men and 30 healthy women (average

age of 33), half of whom were smokers. The participants were randomized to consume their usual diet or receive the addition of a bowlful (85g) of raw watercress each day for eight weeks.

After a seven week period, in which no watercress was consumed, the subjects switched regimens for a further eight weeks. Fasting blood samples were collected at the beginning and end of each eight-week phase of the trial and several measures of lymphocyte DNA damage assessed. Plasma lutein, retinol, alpha-tocopherol and beta-carotene levels were also measured.

The researchers found that significant reductions in DNA damage occurred when the participants consumed watercress. These reductions were found to be greatest among those participants who were smokers.

In addition to reducing DNA damage in the white blood cells (lymphocytes), watercress consumption was also associated with a 9.4 per cent reduction in DNA damage to lymphocytes when challenged with free-radical (cancer-causing toxins) generating hydrogen peroxide. Better still, plasma lutein levels were found to double following the consumption of watercress, and beta-carotene concentrations rose by approximately one third.

The researchers believe that watercress may exert its protective effect on the genes due to its rich antioxidant content – in particular, lutein and beta-carotene. Analysis of watercress leaves detected several beneficial phenolic components such as rutin, as well as a number of glucosinolates, which may also contribute to its protective effect. The difference in beta-carotene levels between smokers and non-smokers in this study could be due to a greater requirement of the vitamin by individuals who smoke.

Commenting on the findings, lead researcher Professor Ian Rowland said: "Our findings are highly significant. Population studies have shown links between higher intakes of cruciferous vegetables like watercress, and a reduced risk of a number of cancers. However, such studies don't give direct information about causal effects. What makes this study unique is it involves people eating watercress in easily achievable amounts, to see what impact that might have on known bio-markers of cancer risk, such as DNA damage. Most studies to date have relied on tests conducted in test tubes or in animals, with chemicals derived from cruciferous vegetables.

"Blood cell DNA damage is an indicator of whole body cancer risk, and, the results support the theory that consumption of watercress is linked to an overall reduced risk of cancer at various sites in the body."

- ## Soya – boosting your intake could reduce your risk of breast and prostate cancer

Soya is one of nature's most magnificent foods, offering a multitude of health benefits – most notably protection against certain cancers, especially breast cancer. Plant chemicals called isoflavones are thought to be largely responsible for soya's health-giving properties. And recent research shows that its beneficial effects extend to managing prostate cancer too.

It is no wonder then that the ancient Chinese dubbed soya the 'miracle bean', whilst in Japan it was revered as one of the five sacred grains (alongside rice, barley, millet and wheat.)

In addition to its anti-cancer effect, soya helps maintain blood levels of insulin and sugar – particularly advantageous for diabetics – at stable levels throughout the day.

Soya is hugely versatile and is available as milk, sausages, nuggets, mince tomiso (fermented bean paste) and tofu – there's a soya source to suit everyone. Unlike most sources of plant protein – pulses, seeds, nuts, grains and other seeds – soya contains an adequate supply of essential amino acids, the building blocks of protein.

Active ingredients found in soya show promise against breast cancer

The active isoflavones in soya are genistein and daidzein. Genistein appears to be effective in helping to slow the progression of prostate cancer, while daidzein plays a therapeutic role in inhibiting the progression of hormone-sensitive breast cancers. It does this by blocking oestrogen-receptor sites on breast cells.

In addition, two non-nutritive compounds in soyabeans, protease inhibitors (enzymes) and phytic acid, have an anti-carcinogenic effect.

Soya contains soluble plant fibre too which binds to toxins, excess oestrogen and cholesterol, mopping them up and excreting them from the body before they can be recirculated.

Soya-rich diet in Japan thought to be responsible for the lowered incidence of prostate cancer

It was epidemiological studies carried out by Dr Stephen Barnes at the University of Alabama in 1996 that first confirmed the link between the consumption of soya foods and a reduced risk of breast, prostate and colon cancer.

These findings backed up studies showing that the incidence of breast, prostate and colon cancers is particularly low in areas of Japan where tofu (made from soya) consumption is high. In fact, levels of these diseases are low throughout Japan in comparison with Western countries, and researchers believe that the levels of isoflavones in the blood are the key to an explanation for this phenomenon.

For example, the Japanese have high isoflavone levels and low rates of prostate cancer (four cases per 100,000 population) and breast cancer (6.6 per 100,000); while here in Britain there are low levels of isoflavones and high rates of prostate cancer (17.1 per 100,000) and breast cancer (27.7 per 100,000).

Preliminary studies indicate a role for genistein in fighting prostate cancer

Now, research carried out by American scientists indicates that the isoflavone genistein is largely responsible for soya's ability to inhibit the progression of prostate cancer.

In a laboratory study conducted by Dr Ralph deVere White and his team at the University of California at Davis, genistein was added to a culture of human prostate cancer cells.

The researchers found that genistein's presence in the culture spurred the production of a gene called p21. This gene is important as it inhibits the manufacture of a protein that helps cancer cells grow. Over time, the prostate cancer cells in the culture began to die off.

In an animal study, the researchers found that genistein was shown to help diminish the size of tumours in cases of prostate cancer *(HealthScout News, June 8 2001)*.

"There is great potential for soya extracts in managing hormone driven cancers such as prostate (and breast) cancer"

Dr Ralph deVere White and his team are now testing the effects of genistein on men suffering from prostate cancer. The scientists hope that the soy extract will have the effect of lowering PSA (prostate specific antigen – an enzyme associated with prostate abnormality) levels.

Tammy Hanna, a nutritional researcher at the University of Kentucky, believes that genistein's anti-carcinogenic properties will prove promising in human trials. "There is great potential for soy extracts in managing hormone-driven cancers such as prostate (and breast) cancer," she says *(Annual Meeting of the American Urological Association, Anaheim, California).*

How to boost your health with soya

There are many delicious soya-based foods to choose from – in the form of soy milk, yoghurts and tofu – all available in supermarkets and health food stores. If 'natural' soya isn't to your taste, you should consider supplementing your diet with Soya Isoflavone tablets. The recommended dosage is one 40mg tablet taken daily with food.

The acrylamide and cancer link

A few years ago Swedish researchers made headlines with a warning that a dangerous compound (most often associated with plastic manufacturing) called acrylamide is created when carbohydrate foods are cooked at high temperatures.

This alarming study was quickly followed up with similar studies in Norway, Switzerland and the UK all of them drawing virtually the same conclusion: Acrylamide, which is known to cause tumours in laboratory animals, is in many prepared foods that our society wolfs down in abundance. French fries, crisps, crackers, pastries, and powdered coffee all contain acrylamide.

• Rosemary is proving an important defence against cancer

Rosemary *(Rosmarinus officinalis)* is a well-known culinary herb. Dried rosemary leaves, whole or ground, are a popular seasoning for food... adding flavour to soups, stews, meat and fish.

Recent research is now revealing even more benefits attached to this remarkable herb, including its ability to help prevent cancer.

The antioxidants contained in rosemary help to protect your body's cells from free radical attack. They include monoterpenes, phenolic diterpenes and flavonoids, which are renowned for their ability to slow down the production of free radicals *(Saen-Lopez R et al. J Chromatogr A 2002953(1-2): 251-256; Lee KG, Shibamoto T. J Agric Food Chem 2002; 50(17): 4947-4952)*. It is also a rich source of vitamin E (alpha tocopherol), another potent antioxidant, which contributes to its free radical fighting powers further still *(Torre J et al. J Chromatogr A 2001; 919(2): 305-311)*.

DNA is your genetic blueprint, and it is particularly prone to injury caused by free radicals. Left unchecked, this damage can eventually lead to cells proliferating out of control, which greatly increases the risk of cancer.

Scientists from the department of Mutagenesis and Carcinogenesis, Cancer Research Institute of Slovak Academy of Sciences, in the Slovak Republic, have found that rosemary extract can significantly help to protect DNA against free radical damage *(Slamenova D et al. Cancer Lett 2002; 177(2): 145-153)*.

By blocking oestrogen, rosemary helps prevent breast cancer

It is well known that an imbalance of oestrogen hormones in women can contribute to breast cancer and cancer of the uterus. Several conventional drugs such as tamoxifen are aimed at blocking the effects of oestrogen to help reduce this risk. However, tamoxifen can cause a range of unpleasant side effects, including hot flushes, vaginal bleeding, headaches and nausea.

Fortunately, rosemary offers a safe and natural alternative treatment. Dr Zhu and colleagues from the Department of Chemical Biology, State University of New Jersey in the US, found that a 2 per cent concentration of rosemary extract given for three weeks was able to significantly inactivate excess oestrogen. Researchers believe that it works by stimulating liver enzymes, which inactivate oestrogen hormones like oestrone and oestradiol *(Zhu BT et al. Carcinogenesis 1998: 19(10): 1821-1827).*

• Include more olive oil in your diet

The benefits of following a Mediterranean-style diet – rich in olive oil as well as cereals, wine, fruits, nuts, legumes, whole grains and fish – just seem to get better and better. Most of the research up until now has concentrated on the well-documented heart-protective benefits that the diet provides.

Now a new study carried out by researchers from five different European countries has concentrated on one vital aspect of the diet – olive oil. They have found that the greater intake of olive oil in Southern European countries may be responsible for the lower rates of cancer observed among individuals living there, in comparison with their Northern European neighbours *(The Journal of the Federation of American Societies for Experimental Biology, January 2007).*

The research team led by Dr Henrik E. Poulsen, of Rigshospitalet, Denmark gave volunteers from Denmark, Finland, Germany, Italy, and Spain 25 millilitres of olive oil each day for three weeks. Urine samples were then analyzed for levels of the waste by-products of cellular oxidative damage, which is a precursor of cancer. While the by-products were higher among Northern European participants at the beginning of the trial, a significant reduction was observed by the study's end.

Commenting on the findings, Dr Poulsen said: "Determining the health benefits of any particular food is challenging because it involves relatively large numbers of people over significant periods of time. In our study, we overcame these challenges by measuring how olive oil affected the oxidation of our genes, which is closely linked to development of disease. This approach allows us to determine if olive oil or any other food makes a difference. Our findings must be confirmed, but every piece of evidence so far points to olive oil being a healthy food."

But frying at high temperatures for long periods causes any fat, and the food fried in it, to break down and produce toxic and cancer-causing chemicals. Quick stir-frying is much healthier.

• Mediterranean diet cuts breast cancer risk in older women

The findings of a French study, published in the October issue of the *American Journal of Epidemiology*, add more evidence to support the anti-cancer benefits of following a Mediterranean diet.

According to the researchers, the incidence of breast cancer may be lowered in postmenopausal women through following a diet comprising mostly of fruits, vegetables, fish and olive/sunflower oil.

The research was initiated in 1990 and involved 65,374 women living in France who were born between 1925 and 1950. Participants completed biennial self-assessment follow-up questionnaires on their health status, medical history, and lifestyle. Dietary data was collected via a self-assessment diet history questionnaire assessing consumption of 208 foods and beverages.

During the study researchers considered potential interactions with known risk factors for breast cancer such as age, educational level, geographic area, body mass index, height, family history of breast cancer, pregnancy and breastfeeding history and the use of vitamin/mineral supplements.

The results showed that after a follow-up period of 10 years, among the women studied, 2,381 developed postmenopausal invasive breast cancer. The researchers said that their findings indicate that a Mediterranean diet is associated with a reduced risk of breast cancer only if food intake remains within recommendations and if 'unhealthy' foods are not consumed in large quantities. They also stated that the risk associated with the 'alcohol/Western' diet (meat products, chips or fries, appetizers, rice/pasta, potatoes, pulses, pizza/pies, canned fish, eggs, alcoholic beverages, cakes, mayonnaise, and butter/cream) was higher in the case of tumours that were oestrogen receptor-positive/progesterone receptor-negative.

Other points noted by the researchers in light of this study are:

- It was difficult to determine which components of the Mediterranean pattern explain the inverse association with breast cancer risk.
- Up to now evidence for associations between breast cancer risk and specific foods or nutrients has been limited, except for alcohol.

Finally, the researchers added that breast cancer incidence varies widely between countries, and that this suggests there may be an influence of environmental factors. As an example, they highlighted that traditionally Japanese women have a low risk of breast cancer but breast cancer incidence in Japan has recently increased alongside major changes in traditional habits, such as diet.

The researchers believe that the increasing incidence of breast cancer in Japan can be attributed (at least partly) to the adoption of a Western diet, which is notably characterized by higher intakes of meat, dairy products, and saturated fat, and decreased consumption of traditional Japanese foods such as seafood products.

• Why an apple a day could keep pancreatic cancer at bay

Research findings from the University of California Los Angeles (UCLA) in the US, have revealed a potential new weapon in the war against pancreatic cancer, one of the deadliest forms of the disease.

Each year about 6,700 people in the UK are diagnosed with pancreatic cancer – and for most, by the time it's detected, there's little that can be done. Pancreatic cancer is often considered a silent disease – hard to detect and diagnose, and nearly impossible to treat, unless it is caught very early. That's what makes prevention efforts all the more important.

There are steps you can take to avoid pancreatic cancer. Modifying lifestyle factors like cigarette smoking and obesity can significantly decrease your risk of pancreatic cancer. Now, according to the latest research findings, grabbing a Granny Smith when you're looking for a snack may be a good idea too.

The study, published in the *International Journal of Cancer*, reports that a specific antioxidant compound found in apples slowed the growth and curbed the spread of pancreatic cancer cells in mice.

Of course, further studies will be required to determine if the compound can treat or prevent cancer in humans, but the results of this study take a promising first step in that direction.

Antioxidants to the rescue... once again

The UCLA researchers decided to examine the preventative effects of natural antioxidants on pancreatic cancer. They knew that quercetin, a powerful antioxidant found in apples, had shown promising cancer-fighting potential against other types of cancer. So they set out to determine how quercetin and three other food-derived compounds might impact on pancreatic cancer.

Their study was divided into two phases. The first measured the effects of quercetin on pancreatic cancer in a strain of mice specially bred to have no immune system. Human pancreatic cells were introduced into the mice, and cancer cells were injected.

Mice treated with quercetin survived an average of 34 per cent longer than untreated mice. The quercetin effectively inhibited the spread of malignant cells and triggered apoptosis, a series of reactions that cause cancer cells to self-destruct.

The second phase of their study investigated the effects of several different plant-based polyphenols on pancreatic cancer cells. Rutin, found in green tea; trans-resveratrol, found in grapes and wine; genistein, found in soybeans; and quercetin were each combined with pancreatic cancer cells in a laboratory.

Except for rutin, all of the polyphenols exhibited potent cancer-fighting properties. In both phases, the researchers concluded that polyphenol antioxidants like quercetin could inhibit pancreatic cancer growth.

- **Could a curry offer effective protection against colon and breast cancer?**

Curcumin, the pungent yellow pigment found in turmeric (an ingredient of curry powder), has a fairly lengthy history as a possible anti-cancer agent. Curcumin appears to be especially effective against breast and colon cancer – two of the leading causes of death from cancer in the Western world. Better still, recent scientific reports have concluded that curcumin is a safe, non-toxic anti-cancer agent *(Curr Pharm Des 2002) 8(19); 1695-1706)*.

In Asian countries, people who consume a lot of turmeric in their diets have been found to have a particularly low incidence of cancer of the bowel, which scientists have attributed to the anti-cancer effects of curcumin.

The mechanism by which curcumin attacks cancer cells is now finally being understood by scientists. It appears to work by blocking certain chemicals which encourage the spread of cancer, such as cytochrome P450, cyclo-oxygenase. This action helps slow the growth of cancer cells until they stop completely – a process referred to in scientific circles as the 'G2 phase arrest'.

Another way curcumin works is by blocking the formation of new arteries, which feed cancerous cells and promote their growth. By restricting these arteries, curcumin is responsible for starving cancer cells and their eventual death *(Bioorg Med Chem 2002, 10(9): 2987-2992).*

Other research shows that curcumin interferes with the enzyme telomerase, which repairs the DNA of cancerous cells. Without an active DNA, cancer cells simply die *(Cancer Lett 2002, 184(1): 1-6).* Amazingly, curcumin is able to distinguish between cancerous DNA material and healthy DNA – destroying the former and leaving healthy DNA intact. Finally, curcumin blocks certain growth factors called kinases, which stimulate cancer cells to develop and multiply.

Curcumin helps switch off breast cancer genes

An animal study has shown that curcumin, prevents breast cancer from spreading to the lungs *(Cell Physiol Biochem 2007; 19: 137-152).*

Scientists at the Anderson Cancer Center in Houston, Texas, have found that curcumin blocks the action of a protein called "nuclear factor Kappa B" which "switches on" the genes that allow breast cancer to develop and grow.

Specifically, curcumin appears to be able to prevent the uncontrolled growth of breast tumour cells, to restore the normal mechanism by which cells die and to prevent cancer spread (metastasis) through the bloodstream and lymphatic system *(Clin Cancer Res 2005; 11: 7490-7498).*

Research also suggests that curcumin can help interfere with the growth factor of signalling pathways in both androgen-dependent and androgen-independent prostate cancer cells *(Mol Urol, 2000; J Biol Chem, May 2000).*

Take 500mg to 1,000mg of curcumin a day.

• Oily fish can help cut colorectal cancer risk

A new study has found that regular and long-term consumption of omega-3 fatty acids and oily fish can slash the risk of developing colorectal cancer by up to 40 per cent.

Over an impressive 22 years of study, both omega-3 and fish intake were associated with cancer risk reduction in the colon and rectum, according to findings by researchers from Harvard and Columbia University.

Megan Hall and her fellow researchers followed 21,376 men participating in the Physicians' Health Study (PHS) trial (started in 1982) for an average of 22 years. The men's intake of fish, and subsequently omega-3 fatty acid intake, was calculated from an abbreviated food-frequency questionnaire.

Over the course of the study, 500 cases of colorectal cancer were diagnosed. In terms of fish intake, the highest average intake was associated with a 40 per cent reduction in the risk of colorectal cancer. In addition, this link was relevant for both colon and rectal cancers.

When the scientists focused on omega-3 fatty acid consumption, they found similar associations, with the highest intakes linked to a 26 per cent reduction in colorectal cancer risk, compared to the lowest average intake.

Commenting on the findings Hall said: "Our results from this long-term prospective study suggest that intakes of fish and long-chain n-3 fatty acids from fish may decrease the risk for colorectal cancer".

Different omega-3, different effects

A study published last year in the *American Journal of Epidemiology (Vol. 166, pp. 1116-1125)* reported that different omega-3 fatty acids conferred different levels of protection. Indeed, increased intake of eicosapentaenoic acid (EPA) was associated with a 41 per cent reduction in risk, while docosahexaenoic acid (DHA) was associated with a 37 per cent reduction in risk, comparing highest against lowest average intakes.

It has previously been proposed that omega-3 fatty acids may inhibit the omega-6 arachidonic acid (AA) cascade that has been linked to cancer formation and cell proliferation.

Metabolism of fatty acids produces compounds called prostaglandins, which can be either pro- or anti-inflammatory. The prostaglandins derived from omega-3 fatty acids are said to be anti-inflammatory and may protect against the development of cancer, while prostaglandins derived from omega-6 fatty acids, like AA, are proposed to be pro-inflammatory.

- **Eat more Brazil nuts to keep prostate and breast cancers at bay**

US researchers from Stanford University released study findings in 2001 showing that men with low blood levels of the trace mineral selenium are four to five times more likely to develop prostate cancer than men with normal levels of the mineral *(J Urology 2001; 166: 2034-8)*.

In an earlier 10-year trial, involving over 1,300 people, those taking 200mcg of selenium daily halved their risk of dying from cancers of the prostate, lung, colon and rectum *(J. Am. Med. Assoc. 276(24): 1957-63, 1996)*.

A recent study conducted at the University of Illinois in the US, suggests that Brazil nuts may play a vital role in preventing breast cancer. According to the researchers who conducted the study, this benefit is probably a result of the high amounts of selenium Brazil nuts contain.

Brazil nuts have a very high selenium level, with fish, shellfish and turkey providing good levels too. Selenium supplements are also available – take 200mcg a day.

- **Vitamin B17 – the remarkable, secret nutrient that one doctor claims can lead to "cancer cells dying off like flies!"**

In the kingdom of the Hunzakuts, high up in the Himalayas, people commonly live to be over 100 and, some, incredibly, to 120! Remarkably, no case of cancer has ever been recorded here, a fact which has remained one of the world's greatest medical mysteries – until now.

So what is the Hunzakuts' secret? The key to a long and healthy life it seems lies in the apricot. Or, more precisely, chemicals in the seed of the apricot known as nitrilosides – or Vitamin B17. The Hunza diet is 200 times richer in Vitamin B17 than the average Western diet.

According to its advocates, the truth about this amazing nutrient, and its ability to help prevent and manage cancer, has scandalously been withheld from the public for more than 50 years. And drug companies, who have a vested interest in aggressively promoting their own high-profit cancer drugs rather than explore cheaper nutrient solutions, are largely responsible.

Why your diet could be seriously compromising your health

As long ago as 1952, Dr Ernest Krebs Jnr, a biochemist in San Francisco, advanced the theory that cancer, like scurvy or rickets, was the result of a nutritional deficiency. He identified this missing dietary component as part of the nitriloside family and christened it Vitamin B17 *(Dr Ernest T Krebs Jnr, The Laetriles/Nitrilosides in the Prevention and Control of Cancer [Montreal: The MacNaughton Foundation, n.d.] p16).*

Nitrilosides occur in over 1,200 edible plants and are particularly prevalent in the seeds of fruits in the *Prunus Rosaceae* family, including bitter almond, apricot, blackthorn, cherry, nectarine, peach and plum. Vitamin B17 is also found in maize, sorghum, millet, cassava, linseed and apple seeds.

Unfortunately, the modern diet provides us with no way near the amount of Vitamin B17 we need. Millet, for example, was once the world's staple grain. But it has now been replaced by wheat that contains practically no Vitamin B17. And as our diets have deteriorated, so the cancer rate has moved steadily upwards to the point where, today, one out of every three people in the UK is destined to contract the disease (*G Edward Griffin, World Without Cancer: The Story of Vitamin B17. American Media, March 2000*).

Vitamin B17-rich foods can help protect you against cancer

The high incidence of cancer has been blamed on the fact that it is essentially an age-related disease, and there is more of it being diagnosed because more of us are living longer nowadays. Yet the average life expectancy is just a few years greater than it was four generations ago. Moreover, in those countries where people live longer than in the UK and the US, cancer rates are lower.

The longevity of the Hunzakuts is a case in point. An analysis of their diet has shown that both the fresh and dried apricots – including the seeds and the oil from the seeds – form a significant part of their daily intake (*Allen E. Banik and Renee Taylor, Hunza Land (Long Beach, Calif: Whitehorn, 1960, pp123-124)).*

This supports what we know about other relatively cancer-free native populations in tropical areas, such as South America and Africa, who also eat an abundance of nitriloside-rich foods.

The potent powers of Vitamin B17 can destroy cancer cells whilst leaving healthy cells intact

But exactly how does Vitamin B17 work to fight against cancer? Firstly, it is important to understand the condition itself. Dr Krebs theorised that cancer was a healing process that had gone wrong.

The body is continually producing new cells – known as trophoblasts – to replace damaged tissue. Once the process is complete, enzymes such as trypsin and chymotrypsin, halt the production of new cells. However, if these enzymes are in short supply – for example, if the immune system is compromised in any way – the trophoblasts continue multiplying and a tumour can result. But nature has provided a back-up system in the form of Vitamin B17.

The Vitamin B17 molecule contains two units of glucose, one of cyanide and one of benzaldehyde. A naturally occurring enzyme called glucosidase 'unlocks' the Vitamin B17 molecule, releasing its component units. The cyanide and benzaldehyde are thought to 'kill' the cancer cell but do not harm healthy cells.

Dr Dean Burk, former head of Cytochemistry at the National Cancer Institute in the US, reported in 1972 that in a series of tests on animal tissue, B17 had no harmful effect on normal cells. However, when Vitamin B17 came into contact with cancer cells, it released large amounts of cyanide and benzaldehyde.

"When we added Laetrile [a medicinal form of Vitamin B17] to a cancer culture… we can see the cancer cells dying off like flies," Dr Burk said (Laetrile Ban May be Lifted, Twin Circle, June 16 1972, p11).

An apple a day has greater implications for your health than previously thought

As modern diets are generally low in Vitamin B17, our natural instinct would be to take it in the form of a dietary supplement. However, Vitamin B17 is available only on prescription as Laetrile. There are several examples of people with cancer who appear to have benefited from treatment with Laetrile to help reduce tumour size (G Edward Griffin, World Without Cancer: The Story of Vitamin B17. American Media, March 2000).

But the greatest benefit of this amazing nutrient is thought to lie in its preventative role, and increasing your dietary intake of Vitamin B17 is believed to be the best way of protecting yourself against the disease.

Dr Krebs strongly recommended a nitriloside-rich diet. For example, he suggested that breakfast might consist of a porridge of buckwheat, millet and flaxseed with stewed prunes. Lima beans with chickpeas for lunch; and a salad with bean and millet sprouts to accompany meat or fish at dinner.

But it requires no small amount of dedication to follow the Krebs' diet – let alone hunt down these foods in your local supermarket! Instead, you can benefit your health simply by eating apricot kernals every day, or grinding them in a blender and using them as a light seasoning for cereals and salads. In fact, you don't actually need a lot of Vitamin B17 to remain healthy. Just eating the seeds from an apple or two a day has important health-giving benefits – apple seeds are a concentrated source of nitrilosides.

For further information read *World Without Cancer: The Story of Vitamin B17*, by G. Edward Griffin (American Media).

- **How a unique form of honey can boost the immune systems of cancer patients undergoing chemotherapy**

Honey has been used medicinally for more than 2,000 years and is known to have potent antibacterial, anti-inflammatory and antioxidant properties *(Bermond P. Biological effects of food antioxidants. Hudson BJF (ed), Food antioxidants, Elsevier, New York, 1990, pp 193-251).*

It can treat a wide range of health problems from coughs, hay fever and stomach upsets to eye problems, skin infections and burns. Its healing properties are thought to come from enzymes that release gluconic acid and hydrogen peroxide.

Now, a particular type of honey, Life Mel Honey, is proving beneficial for cancer patients undergoing chemotherapy and radiation treatment whose immune systems have been seriously compromised.

The honey was originally developed by a Russian microbiologist, Dr Alexander Goroshit, and is now made in Israel where he presently works. His curiosity was initially aroused by the fact that beekeepers' families in a small Russian town remained healthy, despite a local cholera epidemic.

His subsequent research proved that the food bees consume affects their honey's properties *(Kukagawa K, Kunugi A, Kurechi T. Chemistry and implications of degradation of phenolic antioxidants in food antioxidant. Elsevier, New York, 1990).*

So he set about producing honey from bees fed a specific blend of key medicinal herbs – including echinacea, nettles, calendula, *Avena sativa, Melilotus,* Siberian ginseng, red clover, melissa, mulberry, dandelion, chicory, bilberry, elecampane, fig and beetroot. These plants are rich sources of vitamins, minerals, flavonoids and essential oils that work directly on the immune system *(International Conference on Bee Products: Properties, Applications and Aitherapy. Tel Aviv, Israel, May 26-30, 1996).*

Reducing the incidence of neutropenia is vital for the survival of cancer patients

Life Mel Honey has been found to be particularly beneficial against a condition called neutropenia, which cancer patients are especially vulnerable to as a result of chemotherapy.

Neutropenia causes a dangerously low count of neutrophils (infection-fighting white blood cells). Neutrophils usually make up between 50 and 70 per cent of circulating white blood cells and serve as your primary defence against infections by destroying bacteria in your blood.

Patients suffering from neutropenia are far more susceptible to bacterial infections as a result and, without prompt medical attention, their condition can soon become life-threatening. To make matters worse, when a patient's white blood cell count is dangerously low chemotherapy may have to be reduced or discontinued – thereby increasing the risk to the patient from their cancer.

40% of cancer patients suffered no further episodes of neutropenia when taking the honey

A small study by oncologists at Sieff Hospital in Israel has revealed that Life Mel Honey can significantly help reduce the incidence of neutropenia and chemo-induced anaemia *(Medical Oncology, vol 23, no 4, 549-552, 2006).*

The study involved 30 patients, aged 39 to 76, all of whom were either suffering from a primary tumour or metastases (secondary tumour). Cancers included those of the breast, lung and colon. All 30 patients had neutropenia and had been treated with colony-stimulating factors (CSFs).

CSFs are growth factors that stimulate the production of infection-fighting white blood cells. They are often used as a drug treatment for patients with neutropenia but can cause side effects, and in the long run they have been found to make little difference to freedom from infection or to survival rates *(J Clin Oncol, 1998, 16; 3179-3190; Ann Hematol, 1996, 72; 1-9).*

All of the patients were given 5g of Life Mel Honey per day (taken in the morning on an empty stomach) for five days from the start of each chemo treatment. Blood count readings were taken at least once a week after each course of chemo.

The researchers found that 40 per cent of the cancer patients given the honey did not suffer any further episodes of neutropenia and did not require any further treatment with CSFs. In addition, 32 per cent of the patients taking the honey reported "improved quality of life".

Life Mel Honey was also found to be effective at reducing the incidence of chemotherapy-induced anaemia in 64 per cent of the patients. Better still, no side effects were experienced following the use of the honey.

The findings also revealed that Life Mel Honey had a positive effect on the haematopoietic (blood production) system and was able to stimulate the production of white blood cells, red blood cells, haemoglobin and blood platelets.

What to take for best results

The recommended dosage for Life Mel Honey is two teaspoonfuls a day – one in the morning on an empty stomach and one last thing at night. The honey has a pleasant, sweet distinctive taste and although the consistency is thick it dissolves on your tongue quite quickly and pleasantly.

Reports suggest that cancer patients starting Life Mel Honey two weeks prior to receiving treatment experience better results.

Contraindications: Pregnant and breast feeding women should consult their doctor before using Life Mel Honey. The product is not recommended for children under the age of one, or for diabetics or people allergic to bee products.

• Dietary advice that could lower your breast cancer risk

Latest research findings have shown that diet can have a dramatic impact upon the risk of postmenopausal women developing breast cancer. Animal studies have shown that a high intake of saturated fats may increase the risk of breast cancer. Based on this, a research team from the University of Malmö in Sweden devised a study using information gathered on more than 11,000 postmenopausal women.

Researchers followed the women for more than seven years on average, gathering data from diet-history interviews, questionnaires, body measurements and national and regional cancer registries.

When the data was analysed, the Malmö team found that women who had the highest intake of dietary fibre were 40 per cent less likely to develop breast cancer compared with those with the lowest fibre intake. But for women who combined a high fibre diet with a low intake of dietary fats, the risk dropped even more.

In the conclusion to their study, the Malmö authors wrote that, "a dietary pattern characterised by high fibre and low fat intakes is associated with a lower risk of postmenopausal breast cancer."

However, you should make sure you're eating the right kind of fibre to reap the full benefits. Cereal fibre (which is mostly insoluble fibre), such as refined grains, can cause a spike in blood sugar levels. It's no secret that many food products claim to be 'wholegrain' or 'wholewheat,' but actually contain very little of either.

Opt instead for water-soluble fibre:

• Fruits, including oranges, peaches, apples, and grapes
• Vegetables, including carrots, squash, and corn
• Nuts and seeds (in particular, psyllium seeds)
• Legumes, including peanuts, lentils, peas and kidney, black, and pinto beans
• Oats and barley

A number of studies have also shown that a water-soluble fibre called lignan, found in flax seeds, may have a protective effect against breast cancer.

Follow the advice of a leading US doctor...

The Malmö study confirms previous research indicating that a low-fat diet may reduce the risk of breast cancer. But that doesn't mean that any food packaged with a low-fat label is a good choice. And it also doesn't mean that you should avoid high-protein foods.

US physician Dr Jonathan V. Wright believes that specific foods can help prevent breast cancer. Observing that breast cancer risk may be increased by a high intake of saturated fats, omega-6 fatty acids and trans fatty acids, Dr. Wright points out that good amounts of omega-3 fatty acids have been shown to decrease risk.

Dr Wright offers these specific dietary recommendations for lowering breast cancer risk:

- Eat more fish, which is the No. 1 source of cancer-inhibiting omega-3 fatty acids. But to avoid high mercury content, Dr Wright suggests that these fish be avoided: tuna, tilefish, swordfish, shark, king mackerel and red snapper.

- If you can, buy organically raised, 'grass-fed' beef and pork and free-range chicken and turkey. Dr Wright explains that organic and free-range meat contains less omega-6 and much more omega-3 fatty acid content as well as less residue from pesticides, insecticides and herbicides (all of which have been linked to breast cancer).

- Whenever possible, eat organic food. Dr Wright says that if you can't find or afford organic, you can still decrease your breast cancer risk by at least cutting back as much as possible on 'regular' sources of saturated fat and animal protein – mostly the sort you find in supermarkets, such as grain-fed beef, chickens raised in cages, etc.

- Get rid of the margarine! Margarine is made from hydrogenated oil, which is rich in trans fatty acids and omega-6 fatty acids.

- Avoid cow's milk. Studies have shown an association between milk intake and an increased risk of breast cancer. Dr Wright firmly believes that Cow's milk is for calves, not people!

- ## Water helps your body eliminate poisonous waste products

Making sure you eat a healthy, balanced diet – which includes many of the anti-cancer foods featured in this chapter – can help ward off cancer and many other chronic diseases.

However, the importance of drinking adequate amounts of water in addition to following the dietary advice given can't be stressed enough. Water helps to flush harmful toxins from your system. In fact water is more important to the body than any other nutrient and can help prevent many chronic diseases, including cancer.

Yet because water is so commonplace, most people take it for granted and don't drink nearly as much of it as they should to maintain good health. However, unless your body is properly hydrated, you won't experience the full benefits to be had from eating a cancer-preventive diet.

Drinking two litres of water a day is the biggest step you can take to reverse dehydration. To fully re-hydrate your body eat plenty of foods with a high water content such as salad, vegetables, cooked pulses and tofu. However, you should avoid drinking anything other than small sips of water when you are eating in order to facilitate good digestion.

While the merits of water cannot be rated too highly, it is important that you use a water filter or drink bottled water. The reason for this is to help minimise the fluoride content of the water you may be drinking. Fluoridation has been a contentious subject for decades... only now is the full story about this invisible enemy finally emerging.

Fluoride is an odourless, colourless substance but despite these innocent-sounding attributes it is anything but. The fluoride used in water fluoridation projects is actually a toxic by-product of the fertiliser industry.

There are now a growing number of studies linking fluoride consumption to serious conditions such as cancer *(Fluoride 1995; 28(4): 189-92; Fluoride 1996; 29:190-2)*. Research has linked fluoride to as many as 10,000 cancer deaths in the US each year, with a high incidence of bone cancer among men exposed to fluoride.

It's not just water that can be a source of fluoride, it is also present in many toothpastes, mouthwashes, canned foods and even tea bags.

Follow these 7 steps to protect your health against fluoride's harmful effects

1. If you live in a fluoridated area get a reverse osmosis filter fitted to the main kitchen tap. For more information contact The Pure H2O Company on 01784 221188, or visit: www.purewater.co.uk

2. Alternatively, you can help minimise the risk by drinking filtered or bottled water.

3. Use a non-fluoride toothpaste and mouthwash. Fluoride-free toothpaste brands include Boot's Non-Fluoride, Tom's, Tea Tree, and Weleda.

4. Try to be aware of the fluoride content of food and drink – tinned fruit, vegetables and drinks are especially high. Fluoride is present in tea, regardless of whether it's made with fluoridated water or not. So, opt for herbal teas made from non-fluoridated water instead.

5. Eat foods low in fluoride, such as eggs, milk, red meats (not organs), and fruit with protective rinds (such as lemons, bananas and pineapples).

---

6. Supplementing with calcium and magnesium salts helps eliminate fluoride from your body.

7. Avoid using kitchen utensils with non-stick coatings such as Teflon – these are made of fluoride.

Chapter Three: Prostate Cancer

According to Cancer Research UK, prostate cancer is on the increase. With more than 34,000 men diagnosed with it each year, prostate cancer is now the most common type of cancer to affect men in the UK.

The condition kills over 10,000 British men each year and, alarmingly, 50 per cent of men having their prostate gland removed are left impotent *(Cancer Research Campaign Factsheet, 1994)*.

There is no single known cause of the disease, but genetic susceptibility is thought to be a major risk factor *(N Engl J Med 2000; 343(2): 78–85)*. Some prostate cancers are thought to be linked with an increase in levels of the hormone dihydrotestosterone (DHT), which tends to occur as men get older and is also responsible for a much more common, non-cancerous enlargement of the prostate, known as benign prostatic hyperplasia, or BPH.

In fact, your chances of getting prostate cancer increase sharply as you get older – almost 60 per cent of prostate cancer cases are diagnosed in men over 70 years old.

Look out for these warning signs that can spell prostate trouble

As the cancer grows it often causes warning signs because of the prostate gland's strategic position within your body. Your prostate is a small walnut-sized gland located at the base of your bladder that surrounds your urethra – the tube that carries urine from your bladder. Because of its position near the bladder, any enlargement can soon obstruct your urinary flow, causing:

- Frequent need to urinate
- Dribbling after urinating

- Weak urine stream
- Blood in your urine or semen
- A feeling that the bladder has not completely emptied
- Disturbed sleep because of the need to urinate
- Delay or hesitancy before urinating
- Difficult or painful urination or ejaculation

It's important to be aware that these symptoms are also common in non-cancerous conditions, such as infections and BPH – enlargement of the prostate, which affects most men over the age of 65 to some degree.

In cases of advanced prostate cancer, the following symptoms may occur:

- Weight loss
- Bone pain
- Pain in the loins, pelvis or lower back
- Blood in the urine

It's extremely important that you see your doctor straight away if you experience any of the above symptoms.

Could you be at risk?

The causes of prostate cancer aren't yet fully understood. Cases are rare in men aged under 50, however, there are certain things which place some men at higher risk of developing the disease than others:

- Being overweight or obese
- Having a father or brother with prostate cancer
- Being of African-Caribbean or African-American descent and in Western countries
- There is some suggestion that a fat-rich diet may contribute to prostate cancer, but this remains unproven

Studies linking the cancer to vasectomy, an operation to remove a man's fertility, are contradictory.

Time to test your prostate? You need to read this

Your doctor will probably conduct one or more of the following tests to help him make a diagnosis:

A PSA (prostatic specific antigen) blood test can reveal whether you have high levels of this chemical in your blood. PSA is a protein that's naturally produced by the prostate gland. Prostate tumours typically cause an overproduction of PSA, so when a blood test reveals an elevated level of the protein, it's a red flag that warns of possible cancer.

And if elevated PSA were ONLY caused by cancer, then we'd be talking about a truly reliable test. The problem: PSA levels also raise when the prostate becomes infected or when a benign enlargement occurs.

A new study from the Yale School of Medicine in the US, underlines the folly of assuming that the PSA test is anything close to a gold standard for prostate cancer detection.

As reported in a recent issue of *Archives of Internal Medicine*, Yale researchers compared the medical records of about 1,000 subjects; half the men had been diagnosed with prostate cancer and died between 1991 and 1999, and half were men of the same age, chosen at random.

After researchers analysed cases in which subjects had undergone PSA testing and/or digital rectal examination (DRE), they reported that "a benefit for screening was not found" in PSA testing and all-cause mortality.

Even more surprising, when PSA tests were combined with DREs, the results were actually worse.

Digital rectal examination (DRE), involves your doctor inserting a gloved, lubricated finger into your rectum. This allows him to feel your prostate gland through the wall of the rectum and look for any abnormalities. If your doctor discovers any hard or lumpy areas, this indicates that you've got a prostate problem, and more tests will probably be carried out to identify the exact cause of this problem.

PSA test results can vary. Get tested twice!

The Yale researchers concluded that the results of their study "do not suggest that screening with PSA or DRE is effective in reducing mortality."

So are these tried and 'true' methods of checking for prostate cancer worthless? Not at all. But like any tools, their value depends on how they're used.

US healthcare pioneer Dr William Campbell Douglass II, has referred to PSA tests and their follow-up biopsies as "the mainstream's slash-and-burn approach to prostate cancer". But the slashing and burning isn't caused by the test; it's caused by doctors who react inappropriately to the test.

When PSA is elevated, many doctors recommend a biopsy of the prostate; a painful procedure that can result in bleeding and infection. But evidence shows that a great number of these biopsies are completely unnecessary.

In a Memorial Sloan-Kettering Cancer Center study, US researchers tested the reliability of a single PSA result. Over a four-year period, five blood samples were collected from nearly 1,000 men over the age of 60. More than 20 per cent of the subjects were found to have PSA levels that would have prompted many doctors to recommend a biopsy. But half of those men had follow-up tests with normal PSA levels.

The Sloan-Kettering conclusion: A single test that shows an elevated PSA level should be followed with additional screenings to monitor PSA fluctuation.

This research backs up another study in which doctors at the Fred Hutchinson Cancer Research Center estimated that PSA screening resulted in an over-diagnosis rate of more than 40 per cent.

"At present the one certainty about PSA testing is that it causes harm"...

That quote comes from a *British Medical Journal* editorial published over three years ago. And yet some doctors and many men still consider the prostate specific antigen test to be a reliable predictor of prostate cancer.

Dr Chris Hiley of the UK Prostate Cancer Charity recently told *BBC News* that further research is needed to "definitively assess the value of the PSA test".

Let's put that another way, and be very clear so that every man understands what's at stake: A PSA test should not be used as a basis to proceed with invasive procedures that often do more harm than good.

Men take note: Never trust a single PSA test, and never allow a doctor to perform a biopsy based on a single test.

Additional tests that help detect prostate cancer

Imaging techniques may be suggested by your doctor, such as **computerised tomography (CT)**, where a narrow X-ray beam guided by a computer can photograph your prostate to estimate the size of your prostate gland or the presence of a tumour in your prostate.

A **transrectal ultrasound (TRUS)** may also be carried out for further evaluation. A small probe is inserted into your rectum, which uses sound waves to get a better picture of your prostate gland, and inspect it for abnormal conditions like gland enlargement.

Another screening option involves **magnetic resonance imaging**

(MRI), where a scanning technique is used to examine soft body tissue and cells. It helps detect tumours and shows how big they are and if they've spread to other areas of your body.

New test for prostate cancer offers hope in the fight against the disease

Fortunately, a brand new testing procedure looks set to completely revolutionise how prostate cancer is detected.

Researchers from the Jonsson Cancer Center at UCLA, in the US, have just released a report that explains how they created a way to literally light up prostate cancer cells and then find them with special imaging technology.

Their process developed in three steps. First they engineered a virus that recognizes the PSA protein that is only present in prostate cancer cells. In step two the researchers attached luciferase (the substance that creates the glow in fireflies) to the virus which was then injected into tumour-bearing laboratory mice. The virus in effect went looking for the prostate cancer cells, and the luciferase lit them up when they were found.

In the final step they used an advanced, non-invasive imaging technology to not only find illuminated cancer cells, but also to track them as they spread to the lungs and spine. With this imaging technique, the researchers were also able to spot the presence of cancer cells that were still not advanced enough to either trigger symptoms or be detected by conventional methods.

Next step: precise therapy

The UCLA team hopes that in the next step of their research they may be able to attach gene-based therapies to the virus so that they can target and treat only the prostate cancer cells. In a UCLA press release, lead author of the study, Lily Wu, said: "The idea would be to deliver a toxic gene to the cancer that would not harm surrounding healthy cells."

Wu and her colleagues are also confident that it's only a matter of time before they're able to accomplish this same type of prostate cancer cell detection in humans. For human subjects, however, a different sort of imaging system will be required, so another team of researchers at UCLA is already developing the next generation of imaging technology, helped considerably by a huge grant, awarded by the National Cancer Institute.

What conventional treatments are available for prostate cancer?

In working out the best form of treatment for prostate cancer, your doctor will take into account your general health, your age, your expected lifespan, your personal preferences, the anticipated effects of the treatment, as well as the stage and grade (aggressiveness) of your disease.

One of the major difficulties in treating prostate cancer is that no two cancers behave the same. There's the slow-growing cancer that causes no symptoms and doesn't spread. In fact it's normally detected after death if an autopsy is performed. It's been estimated that one in eight men between the ages of 60 and 80 have prostate cancer, but most will never know it. Yet this form of cancer is easily detectable by having simple tests carried out. Then there is the faster-growing, more aggressive form of prostate cancer that spreads early to other tissues and is a major cause of death.

More than one treatment may also be recommended. The most common treatments for prostate cancer include expectant therapy, surgery, radiation therapy, hormone therapy, and chemotherapy. Another option is high intensity focused ultrasound, which uses sound waves to 'melt' away the cancer.

Expectant therapy

Expectant therapy is also called 'watchful waiting', meaning that the prostate cancer is carefully monitored (regular follow-up tests like those already mentioned are carried out) for evidence of cancer progression. No medication is used in this approach. Watching and waiting may be recommended if the prostate cancer is in a very early stage, especially in the cases of older men with small tumours that:

- Are expected to grow very slowly
- Are confined to one area of the prostate
- Are not causing any symptoms or other medical problems

Because prostate cancer cells often spread very slowly, many older men who have the disease live out their normal lifespan without treatment, and without the cancer spreading or causing other problems. Most cancer specialists now agree that, for men with low-grade, localised prostate cancers, a 'wait and see' approach (so-called 'active surveillance') is preferable to aggressive and risky treatments like surgery or radiotherapy.

Prostatectomy

A prostatectomy means that the prostate gland is surgically removed, normally along with small parts of the lymphatic system near the gland. Unfortunately, the operation often causes nerve damage which can make it sometimes impossible for men to achieve an erection afterwards, or maintain complete control over urination.

However, surgeons are learning how to remove the prostate without causing the problematic nerve damage, which was inevitable in the past.

Modern 'nerve-sparing' surgical techniques – combined with impotence treatments – mean that the effects on both sexual function and quality of life can be minimised.

Radiation therapy

Radiation therapy uses X-rays to kill or shrink cancer cells and to decrease their ability to divide and spread. It usually eliminates the need for surgery. Radiation is sometimes used to treat prostate cancer that is still confined to the prostate gland, or has spread only to nearby tissue. If the disease is advanced, radiation may be used to reduce the size of the tumour and to provide relief from symptoms.

Two types of radiation therapy are used:

External beam radiation

This is a painless procedure, which involves the use of a machine to deliver radiation (a high-powered X-ray) to kill cancer cells. While this procedure is normally successful in destroying cancerous cells it can also damage nearby healthy tissue.

However, new techniques have meant that more precise focusing of the radiation can be delivered to your prostate gland without harming surrounding tissue. External beam radiation treatment is normally delivered five days a week (the radiation is only received for about one minute each time) for a total of seven or eight weeks.

The side effects of external radiation for prostate cancer may include diarrhoea, with or without blood in the stool. In rare cases, normal bowel function does not return after treatment is stopped.

Other potential side effects include frequent urination and incontinence (feeling like you have to urinate all the time), burning while urinating, blood in the urine, a feeling of fatigue, which may not disappear until a month or two after treatment stops. In about 30 per cent to 50 per cent of patients, some degree of impotence (inability to get an erection) may occur within two years of radiation therapy.

Internal radiation therapy

Radiotherapy technology advances mean that far higher doses of radiation can be targeted more precisely on the prostate, killing more cancer cells with fewer treatments. Recent advances include the use of a technique called brachytherapy.

There are two major methods of prostate brachytherapy – permanent seed implantation and high dose rate (HDR) temporary brachytherapy. Permanent seed implants involve injecting approximately 100 radioactive seeds into the prostate gland (the implant procedure generally lasts about one to two hours). They give off their cancer-killing radiation at a low dose rate over several weeks or months, and the seeds remain in the prostate gland permanently. Because the seeds used for internal radiation therapy are so small, their presence causes no discomfort, and they are simply left in place.

HDR temporary brachytherapy instead involves placing very tiny plastic catheters into the prostate gland, and then giving a series of radiation treatments through these catheters.

Side effects may include difficulty urinating, pain while urinating, and a decrease in the force of the urine stream. The procedure also may result in impotence.

Hormone therapy

Hormone therapy is the basic treatment for patients whose prostate cancer has recurred after treatment or that has metastasised (spread to other parts of the body).

The goal of hormone therapy is to lower the level of the male hormone, testosterone. Produced mainly in the testicles, testosterone causes prostate cancer cells to grow. Reduced testosterone levels serve to make the prostate cancer shrink and become less active. There are several types of hormone therapy:

- **Orchiectomy** – the surgical removal of the testicles to prevent male hormones from stimulating further growth of the prostate cancer.

- **LHRH Analogs** – drugs to decrease the amount of testosterone produced by a man's body. LHRH analogs are injected monthly in your doctor's surgery. Research shows that the drug can lower the level of testosterone as effectively as surgical removal of the testicles. Side effects include hot flushes and growth of breast tissue.

- **Anti-androgens** – substances to block the body's ability to use testosterone. Even after orchiectomy, a small amount of testosterone is still produced in the body and anti-androgens block the body's ability to use testosterone. Anti-androgens are usually used in combination with orchiectomy or LHRH analogs.

Chemotherapy

Chemotherapy is the use of powerful anti-cancer drugs to kill the cancer cells, and is used for patients whose prostate cancer has spread outside of the prostate gland, or for whom hormone therapy has failed. It has shown only limited success in treating advanced cases of the disease, but it may slow tumour growth and reduce pain. Chemotherapy is not effective against early prostate cancer.

The anti-cancer drugs that are given to patients are normally administered intravenously (injected into a vein). The drugs damage cancer cells, but they also damage normal cells and hospitalisation may be needed to monitor the treatment and to control its side effects.

Common side effects include nausea and vomiting, hair loss, anaemia, reduced ability of blood to clot, mouth sores, and increased likelihood of developing infections. Side effects and the degree to which they are experienced differ. However, most side effects disappear once the treatment is stopped.

Safe and effective natural remedies can help you avoid risky surgery

Only a doctor can judge the severity of your prostate cancer and whether a particular treatment is suitable for you. And, whilst these remedies are natural, they can have side effects if mixed with medication.

For this reason, it is extremely important to consult your doctor if you are already on medication or undergoing another treatment for cancer before deciding to take any of the supplements listed, in order to prevent any possible contraindications.

In addition, it is important to realise that there is no telling which treatment, or combination of treatments, will work best for you. While one supplement can produce noticeable improvements in one individual, it may have little or no effect on another person.

Likewise, natural remedies typically take longer to work than conventional drugs. For this reason, you should allow enough time for a supplement to work properly. It may be the case that you have to try a few different treatments before you find one that works for you.

- **Stem the growth of cancerous cells and reduce the size of your prostate with these 4 incredible all-natural remedies:**

1. The bark of *Pygeum africanum* – a large tree that grows at high altitudes in Africa – is a rich source of sterols and other compounds such as triterpenoids, which have been found to reduce swelling and inflammation of the prostate *(Phytotherapy 68(3): 205-218, 1997)*.

Scientists from the Philipps University in Marburg, in Germany, have found that pygeum contains a special chemical called dichloromethane, which prevents the production of testosterone – large amounts of this hormone encourage cancer cells to grow and develop *(Schleich S, Papaioannou M, Baniahmad A, Matusch R. Planta*

Med. 2006; 72(9): 807-13). The recommended dosage for pygeum is 100-200mg a day.

2. Saw palmetto is another rich source of sterols, which block the production of DHT – a potent hormone which stimulates the growth of the prostate gland *(Prostate 43(1): 49-58, 2000; Can Pharm J, 1997: 130(9) 37-44)*. It also blocks the effect of male hormones such as testosterone and relaxes the muscle fibres within the prostate, allowing urine to flow more easily through the urethra. The recommended dosage is 160-240mg of saw palmetto extract, taken twice a day.

3. Another effective remedy against prostate cancer is a member of the carotenoid family called **astaxanthin**. It helps your body produce more immune-boosting chemicals like interferon, which attacks and destroys cancerous cells. The recommended dose is 1mg twice a day.

US researchers from the Research and Development, Triarco Industries, Wayne, have discovered that astaxanthin is far more effective when taken alongside saw palmetto. This combination was found to prevent the spread of prostate cancer by up to 38 per cent *(Anderson ML. J Herb Pharmacother. 2005; 5(1): 17-26)*.

4. Zinc is an essential nutrient for good prostate health. The prostate gland contains more of the trace mineral zinc than any other organ in the body. Supplementing with this mineral can help reduce the symptoms of BPH and help fight prostate cancer too.

Researchers found that zinc prevented cancerous cells from thriving when they incubated human prostate carcinoma cells with zinc – this showed a 50 per cent inhibition of cell growth. The researchers attributed decreased cell growth to apoptosis (programmed cell death), concluding that the inability to retain high zinc levels is an important factor in the development and progression of malignant prostate cells *(Prostate 1999; 40 (3): 200-207)*.

Take 60mg of zinc a day for the first six months, then reduce to 15-30mg a day. Vitamin B6 is essential for the proper absorption of zinc, so take 50mg of this nutrient at the same time.

- **How a blend of the most powerful plant antioxidants – contained in a tasty new drink – can help you fight prostate cancer**

A brand new, all-natural product called Dr Red Blueberry Punch – which contains a unique blend of plant extracts and 'superfoods', including concentrated extracts of blueberries, elderberries, raspberries, grape seeds and skins, citrus peel, ginger, olives and olive leaves, turmeric and green tea – has been found to be extremely effective in the fight against prostate cancer.

Impressive research findings have revealed that Dr Red Blueberry Punch, which is available as a cordial, helps reduce pain and inflammation, prevents tumour growth, kills cancerous cells and prevents cancer spreading to other parts of the body.

As a result it holds great promise as a complementary, non-invasive treatment for prostate cancer, which can be used in conjunction with active surveillance or conventional interventions. Not only that but many of the ingredients contained in the formula also have proven benefits for cardiovascular and joint health.

This potent cocktail delivers a knockout blow to cancer cells

New research carried out at the University of Sydney, Australia, has demonstrated that Dr Red Blueberry Punch directly inhibits prostate cancer cell growth *(Singh J, Yao M, Jardine G, Dong Q. Suppressive effects of a phytochemical cocktail on prostate cancer growth in vitro and in vivo. American Association for Cancer Research Conference: Frontiers in Cancer Prevention Research, 5-8 December 2007, Philadelphia, USA).*

This effect was seen both in laboratory tissue cultures and when added to the drinking water of mice that had been inoculated with human prostate cancer cells and had actively growing tumours. Blueberry Punch appears to stop cancer cells developing by blocking the action of a protein called cyclin D1, which promotes their growth.

Human clinical trials using Blueberry Punch with prostate cancer patients have just been completed at Queensland University in Brisbane. Seventy-two men participated in three separate trials, drinking three glasses of Blueberry Punch per day, prior to standard treatment with surgery, radiotherapy or hormone therapy. The results have not been released yet (we've been checking every day right up to the time of going to print), but initial indications appear to be extremely promising.

Research has also been going on around the globe into the ways in which the individual ingredients in Dr Red Blueberry Punch attack prostate cancer. US scientists at the University of Illinois have looked at the effects of blueberry extract (a rich source of proanthocyanidins – part of a group of plant chemicals called flavonoids) on prostate cancer cells. They found that cells from tumours that were sensitive to male sex hormone (androgen) levels were inhibited by the blueberry extract and their proliferation was significantly reduced *(Cancer Lett 2006; 231: 240–246)*.

Other studies have found that a flavonoid called hesperidin, which is present in the peel of citrus fruits – another ingredient in the formula – has the same effect of reducing cell growth in androgen-dependent prostate cancers. It appears to work by interfering with the androgen receptor sites and chemical signalling pathways that promote cell proliferation *(Phytother Res 2009 Jun 22. [Epub ahead of print])*.

Proanthocyanidins in elderberry juice have also been found to inhibit the proliferation of prostate cancer cells in laboratory experiments; and resveratrol, from red grape skins, suppressed the development of prostate cancer in animal experiments, by reducing both cancer cell proliferation and the production of a cancer growth factor called IGF-1 *(Anticancer Res. 2007 Mar-Apr; 27(2): 937-48; Mol Oncol 2007; 1(2): 196-204).*

Green tea and grape extracts help block tumour development and metastasis

In order for prostate cancer cells to reproduce and form a tumour, they need to make copies of their DNA (deoxyribonucleic acid, which holds the genetic blueprint for a cell's development and functioning). When US scientists, at the University of South Florida, treated mice with compounds called catechins, derived from green tea, they found that this process was blocked due to reduced production of a chemical called DNA replication factor MCM7 *(Prostate 2009; 69(15): 1668-1682).*

In a process called apoptosis, also known as 'cell suicide', cancer cells can be triggered to play an active role in their own death. Newly-published research from the Republic of Korea has revealed that a compound present in grapes, called piceatannol, induces apoptosis in human prostate cancer cells *(J Med Food. 2009 Oct; 12(5): 943-51).* Apoptosis of prostate cancer cells has also been shown to be triggered by a flavonoid called quercetin, present in red grapes, raspberries, citrus fruits and green tea – all of which are ingredients in Blueberry Punch *(Oncol Res 2006; 16(2): 67-74).*

In order for a prostate cancer tumour to grow rapidly, it needs to establish its own blood supply – a process called angiogenesis. Scientists at the University of Winsconsin, in the US, have discovered that an extract of green tea can block this process by reducing the expression of genes that produce angiogenesis-stimulating growth factors *(J Nutr 2003; 133(7 Suppl): 2417S-2424S).* In the same research, green tea extract was found to inhibit the spread of cancerous cells from prostate tumours to other parts of the body (metastasis), again by suppressing the expression of the relevant genes.

What to take for best results

Dr Red Blueberry Punch comes as a concentrated cordial. The recommended dose is 25ml to 75ml daily, diluted 1:6 with water. If you have been diagnosed with prostate cancer, or if you are taking warfarin or other blood-thinning drugs, you are advised to talk to your doctor before taking Blueberry Punch.

- **Healthy Cells Prostate™ helps maintain the health of your prostate and reduces your risk of prostate cancer**

Studies have shown that natural remedies can play a beneficial role in the fight against prostate cancer. It's refreshing to discover that the research charity Prostate UK recommends certain supplements, including selenium and lycopene, to help prevent prostate disease *(http://www.prostateuk.org/research/research.htm)*.

Now these two nutrients, together with other carefully selected and clinically-proven ingredients – including calcium D-glucarate, broccoli extract, maitake mushroom and green tea – are available in an exciting new formula called Healthy Cells Prostate™.

It acts as a powerful defence against prostate problems by promoting the development of healthy prostate cells, improving prostate function, boosting immunity and encouraging your body's detoxification process.

Calcium D-glucarate helps rid your body of cancer-causing substances

One of the main active ingredients in Healthy Cells Prostate™ is calcium D-glucarate. This compound is converted in your stomach to glucaric acid, which helps eliminate harmful chemicals and excess steroid hormones from your body and protects your prostate from their adverse effects.

One of the key ways in which your body gets rid of toxic chemicals and excess hormones is by combining them with glucuronic acid in your liver, and then excreting them in your bile. However, this process can be compromised by an enzyme called beta-glucuronidase, which is produced by certain bacteria that reside in your gut. This enzyme breaks the bond between the toxic compound and glucuronic acid, and this releasing action means that these toxic chemicals can then be easily reabsorbed into your body to cause harm, instead of being excreted.

Fortunately, calcium D-glucarate is able to reduce the activity of beta-glucuronidase – allowing your body to eliminate various toxic chemicals and hormones that might otherwise contribute to cancer development. High levels of beta-glucuronidase are associated with an increased risk of hormonally-sensitive cancers of the prostate and breast *(Cancer Detect Prev. 21: 178-190. 1997; Carbohydr Res.105: 95-109. 1982; Hepatology 9: 552-556. 1988; FASEB. 5: A930. 1991).*

Healthy Cells Prostate™ also contains broccoli extract, which is another excellent source of glucaric acid, as well as the cancer-fighting compounds indole-3-carbinol and sulforaphane.

The mushroom that helps prevent the spread of abnormal prostate cells

Another ingredient in Healthy Cells Prostate™ is maitake mushroom – or more specifically a pure extract called D-fraction, which contains a concentration of the mushroom's immune-activating component.

Studies have revealed that maitake contains a polysaccharide, or carbohydrate, called beta glucan that appears to activate your immune system's 'soldiers' that travel your bloodstream.

One of these is a large white blood cell called a macrophage which swallows microorganisms, pathogens and tumour cells. This action has important implications for fighting cancer and the latest published research on maitake mushroom D-fraction reveals that the mushroom has the ability to initiate the death of prostate cancer cells (*Journal of Hematology & Oncology. 1: 25. 1-8. 2008*).

Lycopene and selenium – a powerful duo in the fight against prostate cancer

Healthy Cells Prostate™ also contains lycopene – the pigment that causes the red colour in tomatoes. As mentioned on page 25, this powerful antioxidant has been found to play a major role in maintaining the health of the prostate gland and research suggests that lycopene supplements could reduce the growth of prostate cancer (*J Natl Cancer Inst. 94(5): 391-391. 2002; Cancer Epidemiol Biomarkers Prev 2001; 10: 861-8*).

Patients scheduled for prostate removal received a 15mg lycopene supplement twice a day for three weeks. They experienced an average 20 per cent drop in prostate specific antigen levels – a diagnostic measure for prostate cancer – and their tumours began to shrink.

The mineral selenium has been added to the formula because of its remarkable ability to help prevent prostate cancer. Researchers at Stanford University in the US found that men with low blood levels of the trace mineral selenium are four to five times more likely to develop prostate cancer than men with normal levels of the mineral (*J Urology 2001; 166: 2034-8*).

In an earlier 10-year trial, involving over 1,300 people, those taking 200mcg of selenium daily halved their risk of dying from cancers of the prostate, lung, colon and rectum (*J. Am. Med. Assoc. 276(24): 1957-63, 1996*).

Study reveals green tea's cancer-fighting properties

Finally on to why green tea has been included in Healthy Cells

Prostate™. According to a study published in the US journal *Cancer Prevention Research*, a chemical it contains, polyphenon E, appears to be able to slow the progression of prostate cancer.

The study included 26 men, aged 41 to 72 years, who had been diagnosed with prostate cancer and who were scheduled for radical prostate surgery. Patients took four capsules containing polyphenon E – the equivalent of around 12 cups of green tea – for an average of 34 days, up until the day before their surgery.

The study found a significant reduction in levels of hepatocyte growth factor (HGF), vascular endothelial growth factor (VEGF), and prostate specific antigen (PSA) – all markers of prostate cancer – with some patients demonstrating reductions of more than 30 per cent.

What to take for best results

The recommended dosage for Healthy Cells Prostate™ is one tablet taken twice a day with meals, or as otherwise directed by your healthcare practitioner. As always, it is important you consult your doctor prior to using the supplement if you are currently on any medication.

Increase your intake of pomegranates to protect your prostate

When pomegranate juice was given to prostate cancer patients with rising levels of PSA ('prostate specific antigen' – a marker for the progress of the disease), scientists found that it significantly increased the time taken for PSA levels to double, from 14 to 26 months on average *(Clin Cancer Res 2006; 12(13): 4018-4026)*.

In an animal study, pomegranate extract was found to significantly reduce the growth rate of human prostate cancer tumours in mice *(J Agric Food Chem 2007; 55(19): 7732-7737)*.

- ## How a mushroom heralds an important breakthrough for prostate cancer sufferers

The Chinese mushroom Lingzhi *(Ganoderma lucidum)* has long been held in high esteem in China as a potent natural remedy, which is also thought to be capable of bestowing longevity. In fact, ancient Chinese holy men believed that whoever consumed the mushroom regularly would become immortal, which is why they coined it, 'the mushroom of immortality'.

Now, while this mushroom certainly won't make you live forever, scientists have been investigating the medicinal properties of Ganoderma and have been astounded by the results yielded so far.

They've been particularly impressed by the powerful anti-cancer action ganoderma appears to possess. Numerous studies, including one carried out at the Department of Medical Biochemistry, Ehime University in Japan, have revealed that it can help prevent the spread of cancer, especially of the prostate, breast, liver and spleen *(Kimura Y, Taniguchi M, Baba K. Anticancer Res 2002; 22(6A): 3309-3318).*

Ganoderma encourages the death of cancerous cells

According to Japanese researchers, ganoderma contains natural chemicals called triterpenoids, which possess an important anti-cancer action. They are able to inhibit the blood supply to cancerous cells – preventing oxygen and other nutrients from feeding them *(Kimura Y, Taniguchi M, Baba K. Anticancer Res 2002; 22(6A): 3309-3318).*

On the other side of the Pacific, US scientists working at the Cancer Research Laboratory, Methodist Research Institute in Indianapolis, have shown that ganoderma is able to block several chemicals, including AP-1, NF-kappaB and uPA, which promote the spread and development of cancerous cells *(Sliva D, Labarrere C, Slivova V, Sedlak M. Biochem Biophys Res Commun 2002; 298(4): 603-612).*

According to Dr Sliva who led the study: "Our data suggest that the spores and the body of *Ganoderma lucidum* inhibit the spread of breast and prostate cancer cells by a common mechanism, and would have a potential therapeutic use for the treatment of cancer."

Protects DNA and possesses potent anti-inflammatory properties

Scientists have theorised that another possible way in which ganoderma may prevent cells from turning cancerous, is by protecting vital DNA tissue. When DNA becomes damaged by free radicals, toxins or ultraviolet radiation, the risk of cancer is known to increase.

Korean scientists from the Korea Atomic Energy Research Institute tested ganoderma on cancerous cells and then examined the DNA. They found that ganoderma protects DNA from damage caused by free radicals and by radiation. They concluded that the mushroom merits further investigation as a potential preventative agent against cancer *(Kim KC, Kim IG. Int J Mol Med 1999; 4(3): 273-277).*

Natural plant chemicals called phenolic compounds, which are known to be extremely effective in fighting free radicals, are also thought to play an important role in fighting cancer. Chinese researchers from the National Chunh-Hsing University, in Taiwan, have found that ganoderma contains high concentrations of these beneficial phenolic compounds *(Mau JL, Lin HC, Chen CC. J Agric Food Chem 2002; 50(21): 6072-6077).*

Finally, ganoderma appears to inhibit an inflammatory chemical called tumour necrosis factor (TNF). This chemical is strongly implicated in heart disease, diabetes, dementia and cancer. Ganoderma is able to keep TNF under control, which may reduce the risk of these chronic conditions developing *(Gao Y, Zhou S, Wen J. Life Sci 2002: 72(6): 731-745).*

Prostate cancer appears to respond particularly well to ganoderma

A team of scientists from the Department of Urology, College of Physicians and Surgeons of Columbia University in New York, reported on the remarkable case of a patient with prostate cancer.

This patient received treatment with ganoderma and genistein every day for six weeks before he was due to have surgery to remove his prostate. Genistein is a plant chemical present in soya that has been found to help prevent prostate cancer.

This combined treatment approach produced a significant effect on his prostatic specific antigen (PSA) levels. A PSA blood test is commonly performed to evaluate prostate problems, as patients with prostate cancer typically have high PSA levels.

After the six-week treatment programme, doctors were amazed to discover that the patient's PSA reading had fallen from an initial 19.7 ng/mL to a mere 4.2 mg/mL. When the patient went to have his surgery performed, the surgeons found that there was no sign of cancer in his prostate tissue *(Ghafar MA, Golliday E, Bingham J et al. J Altern Complement Med 2002; 8(4): 493-497).*

This is far from being an isolated case. Two years earlier, doctors working at the Squier Urological Clinic, Columbia-Presbyterian Medical Center in New York, reported the recovery of two patients with prostate cancer, who were treated with ganoderma.

Both men had been offered conventional treatment for their prostate cancer but decided to opt for a natural treatment approach instead. In this instance, they received ganoderma together with other herbs like saw palmetto, which has also been found to be effective against prostate cancer.

Again, both patients' PSA readings were found to have dropped significantly. No side effects were reported in either case *(de la Taille A, et al. J Altern Complement Med 2000; 6(5): 449-451).*

What to take for best results

The recommended dosage for maintaining overall health is 0.5g to 1g of ganoderma a day. For those at high risk of cancer (such as those with a family history of the disease) a dosage of 2-5g of Ganoderma is suggested as a preventive measure. No adverse side effects have been reported following the use of ganoderma.

- **Discover the traditional Vietnamese medicine that may hold the key to overcoming prostate and ovarian disorders**

Most people are familiar with traditional Chinese medicine and the inroads it's made as a modern approach to healing. But, less is known about traditional Vietnamese medicine.

One of its most valuable herbs is called *Crinum latifolium*. Apparently, it's so revered in Vietnam that it used to be reserved only for royalty and was known both as the 'Medicine for the King's Palace' and the 'Royal Female Herb'.

Those traditional references actually highlight one of crinum's most unique aspects – its ability to help both sexes by targeting prostate and ovarian problems. Crinum is so established and widely used as a treatment for prostate and ovary diseases in Vietnam that their crops of the herb are generally prohibited from being exported.

That's why we're delighted to introduce Healthy Prostate & Ovary – one of the first crinum products we know of that's available in the UK. As well as crinum it also contains five other herbs – alisma plantagoquatica, astragalus, momordica charantia, carica papaya leaf, and annona muricata leaf – all known for their immune- and energy-boosting effects.

Promising results in the fight against prostate cancer

Although most of the research on crinum focuses on men, it all started when the Hoang family studied its effect on ovarian health. Dr Kha Hoang was the chief teacher and medical doctor for the Vietnamese royal family. In 1984 his daughter had so many cysts on one of her ovaries that surgery was planned to remove it. Dr Hoang gave her a tea made with crinum leaves to drink, and about six weeks later the cysts were gone.

Today, three generations of the Hoang family are integrated medicine practitioners. The family has used crinum together with other supportive herbs in treating a variety of prostate and ovarian conditions. Biopsies confirmed 16 cases of advanced prostate cancer were completely cured regardless of prostate specific antigen (PSA) levels. In fact, sometimes PSA levels go up in men taking crinum, even though testing shows that their prostate cells are normal and healthy.

That is exactly what happened to Ken Malik, the co-founder and Executive Director of the Prostate Awareness Foundation, a non-profit organisation based in San Francisco in the US. In his own battle with prostate cancer, Malik chose to take the natural approach – opting for a therapeutic regimen of nutrition and exercise. He also used the herbal supplement PC SPES for eight years and found doing so stabilised his condition.

PC SPES was a herbal formula that showed remarkable results in treating prostate problems. However, a few years ago, it was pulled from the market after researchers discovered that some PC SPES products claiming to be all-natural actually contained synthetic, potentially harmful substances. Malik began his search for a replacement, which led him to crinum.

92.6% success rate when it comes to reducing BPH symptoms

Malik started taking crinum in January 2002, and, over the course of the next 10 months, his PSA actually increased. Most of the time, this would be cause for concern. But Malik's most recent biopsy showed only healthy tissue. His experience might add some support to recent reports that claim the PSA test might not be the best indicator of prostate cancer risk. Malik was excited enough about his own experience to organise a small informal trial with 10 members of the Prostate Awareness Foundation.

Participants were told to take nine crinum tablets each day for three months. All 10 noted some kind of functional improvement. Not everyone experiences elevated PSA levels using crinum. Sometimes its benefits follow a more predictable path, like the testimonial from a 58-year-old man who had a PSA of 93 when he went to his urologist for treatment.

He'd waited so long that his cancer had spread to his bones, intestines, and lymph nodes. He was placed on an aggressive herbal programme that included crinum. After just four months, his PSA was down to 0.9 and the symptoms he'd been experiencing – difficulty urinating, swelling in his legs, and extreme fatigue – had all disappeared.

Crinum can also help alleviate the symptoms of benign prostatic hyperplasia (BPH) – an enlarged prostate. The main symptom of BPH is frequent and sometimes painful urination. There are over 500 individual case histories of successful crinum treatment for BPH. And after seven years of research, the International Hospital in Vietnam reported that 92.6 per cent of patients had good results using crinum for BPH (confirmed by measurements of prostate size and clinical evaluation by urologists) *(The Journal of Health Ministry of Vietnam, December 20, 2002, N 207).*

Boosts immunity by encouraging your cells to communicate

Researchers believe crinum works at the simplest level – your cells. In order for your body to function properly, all of those cells must communicate.

Cells communicate with one another to determine the correct balance of cell proliferation and apoptosis, or death. Basically, they're constantly working together to regulate how many cells you have – and how healthy they are – at any given moment.

But if your cells aren't communicating properly, apoptosis may not happen the way it should, which means that unhealthy, even cancerous, cells can continue to thrive and mutate. Recent experiments show that crinum extract helps cells produce a substance called neopterin, which they send out to communicate with immune cells, calling them into action against cancer and other foreign invaders *(Int Immunopharmacol. 2001 Nov; 1(12):2143-50).*

What to take for best results

The recommended dosage for Healthy Prostate & Ovary is three 600mg tablets taken three times a day. If you're battling cancer or any other serious illness, it is important that you consult your doctor before using this product.

- **Wipe out prostate cancer without touching a single healthy cell? An incredible new breakthrough looks set to do just that**

A ground-breaking new formula is fast proving its worth in the fight against prostate cancer. It has been found to repair DNA damage that, left unchecked, can cause cancer; it also attacks cancerous cells while leaving healthy cells intact.

Prostabel is a truly remarkable breakthrough that owes its existence to a brilliant scientist who was far ahead of his time.

You might remember the names Watson and Crick from science classes. Back in the early 1950s, they described the double-helix structure of DNA, the very blueprint of our bodies. But around that same time, a young biochemist and biologist was going farther – much farther – at the prestigious Pasteur Institute in Paris.

Dr Mirko Beljanski devoted his entire life to studying cell regulation and replication, especially how DNA and RNA take part in cellular health. Your DNA holds your unique genetic code, and RNA controls what happens with the cells in your body.

Beljanski was especially interested in what happens when something goes wrong with cell regulation – and how to get it back on track. He discovered that before genetic mutations of DNA occur, attacks on the double helix itself create a structure that no longer functions properly. This allows damaged DNA to replicate much faster, gaining speed with each division. Beljanski connected this excess replication and increased cell multiplication to cancer.

He knew he was on to something and theorised that if he could find a way to stabilize that second structure, he could prevent DNA from abnormally replicating and causing cancer. So he started a tireless search for natural substances that could stabilize DNA without harmful side effects.

Ancient remedies reinvented as modern cancer-fighters

This led him to *Pao pereira* and *Rauwolfia vomitoria*, both of which have been used for centuries by indigenous peoples for a variety of ailments. Dr Beljanski discovered that they can actually repair abnormal DNA structure.

He demonstrated that, at optimal doses, these two herbs stopped the proliferation of cancer cell lines while sparing healthy cells –

unlike chemotherapy and radiation, which destroy cancer cells and healthy cells without discrimination. This effect was the same against several kinds of cancer – including prostate, brain, colon, liver, kidney and skin cancer *(Genetics and Molecular Biology 2000. 23(1): 29-33).*

Testing *Rauwolfia vomitoria,* he found that, with high doses, up to 80 per cent of mice with cancer that were treated with the extract lived 90 days. Those who went untreated were all dead by day 40. The mice Beljanski deemed cured survived in 'excellent condition' *(Oncology 1986. 43: 198-203).* He went on to use both extracts successfully in numerous human case studies.

Dr Beljanksi wanted to make sure his life's work didn't stop with his death. So before he died in 1998, he entrusted his research to Natural Source, which at the time was a new company devoted to advancing the world of natural medicine.

Their devotion to Beljanski's mission shows in their work. The ingredients in Prostabel are painstakingly harvested from the far reaches of the earth – *Pao pereira* comes from the Amazon Rain Forest, and *Rauwolfia vomitoria* is gathered from the root of a tropical African tree. They're then purified and rigorously tested.

Lowers PSA readings and improves urinary symptoms

The work of Mirko Beljanski – and Natural Source's continuation of that work – caught the eye of Dr Aaron Katz, a leader in the field of natural medicine and men's health.

He set to work studying *Pao pereira* and *Rauwolfia vomitoria,* and the power of these two herbs was revealed almost immediately. In fact, members of Dr. Katz's team have called the two herbs the "most promising candidates to date" when it comes to fighting prostate and bladder cancer.

A trial of 30 men with high PSA readings (a marker for prostate cancer) and a negative biopsy (meaning they don't have cancer yet) showed that Protabel significantly lowered PSA over the course of a year.

And the men taking Prostabel had other good news to report – a dramatic improvement in urinary symptoms. They had better streams and better flow rates, and weren't getting up as often at night. Better still, no side effects were experienced.

Peter Williams, who was diagnosed with adenocarcinoma (cancer originating in glandular tissue) at the age of 68, wrote to Natural Source to tell them about the remarkable success he experienced after using Dr Beljanski's formula. His PSA dropped from 5.57 to 0.10, and his radiologist can't find anything abnormal. He's been in remission for two years, with his PSA holding steady.

A major human trial to assess Prostabel's cancer-fighting potential is currently underway at Columbia's Department of Urology, and preliminary results are very promising.

Cancer cell growth cut by 90% in less than a day

Overall, research has shown that *Pao pereira* extract more potently induces cell death than the *Rauwolfia vomitoria* extract. But the Rauwolfia extract is more successful at inhibiting cell cycle progression of prostate cancer cells – meaning it hampers their ability to grow and divide. Together, in Prostabel, they're a formidable force against prostate cancer.

In an in-vitro study, *Pao pereira* was added to a line of cultured prostate cancer cells. The extract was found to significantly suppress cell growth – by 90 per cent as early as 24 hours after exposure! – and caused cancer cells to die. It also caused a significant decrease in overall tumour size.

Surprisingly, the greatest effect on tumour growth occurred at the lower doses of *Pao pereira* tested on mice. At doses of 10 and 20mg/kg per day, tumour volume was reduced by 80 per cent and 75 per cent, respectively. Because *Pao pereira* has tumour-suppressing activity without toxicity, it may act as a safe and effective preventative against prostate cancer *(Journal of the Society for Integrative Oncology 2009. 7(2): 59-65).*

And *Rauwolfia vomitoria* is just as impressive. In one trial, it was shown to suppress the growth of cancer cells. In another, it decreased tumour volume in mice by 58-70 per cent depending on dose (7.5-75 mg/kg) over a 72-hour period *(Bemis, D.L., et al. Anti-prostate cancer activity of a novel extract from the tropical African shrub, Rauwolfia vomitoria. Columbia University Department of Urology).*

What to take for best results

Take up to 10 capsules per day with a glass of water, or as otherwise recommended by your healthcare practitioner. It is extremely important that you consult your doctor prior to taking Prostabel, especially if you're already on any medication.

Chapter Four: Breast Cancer

Separating myth from fact to help protect you against the disease

B reast cancer is the most common form of cancer in the UK – approximately 46,000 people are diagnosed every year and, in fact, every 11 minutes someone is diagnosed with the disease. One in every nine women in the UK will develop breast cancer at some point in her life, although men can also be affected. Worryingly, the disease is now the main cause of death in women under 55.

Breast cancer has received a lot of media coverage, including conflicting reports over the safety of screening programmes and disturbing new evidence about the link between HRT and breast cancer.

Yet rather than helping to clarify the situation, all these scare stories have succeeded in doing is leaving many women feeling both anxious and confused as to the best way of protecting themselves against this potentially life-threatening condition.

Fortunately, there are safe and effective natural alternatives to help lower your risk of developing the disease. This advice applies to both men and women, as although breast cancer mainly affects women, men (as already mentioned) are at risk from getting it too since both sexes have breast tissue.

Taking HRT could be increasing your risk of breast cancer by up to 40%

While hormone replacement therapy (HRT) may be effective at combating the symptoms of the menopause, its ability to stop hot flushes comes at a high price – an increased risk of breast cancer.

A major US study into the effects of HRT, conducted by the National Institutes for Health, was dramatically halted three years before it was due to end after scientists found that it increased the risk of breast cancer, heart attack and stroke.

The US National Cancer Institute has looked at follow-up data from several studies between 1980 and 1995 in which a total of 46,000 healthy women took HRT. It found that women using combined oestrogen-progestogen HRT (as used in the above study) for four years had a 40 per cent higher risk of breast cancer *(JAMA 283: 485-91 & 534-5, 2000)*. Clearly, avoiding HRT and managing your menopause naturally instead is one step you can take to reduce your risk of breast cancer.

Most breast cancer risks relate to a woman's reproductive history. Late menopause, an early first period, late first pregnancy, and few (or no) children are all associated with an increased likelihood of breast cancer. Other risk factors are oral contraceptive use, obesity and high alcohol consumption.

Diet is important, too, as shown in the findings of a recent Harvard study that oriental women who give up their traditional 'soya and vegetable' diet in favour of Western eating patterns increase their breast disease risk by up to 90 per cent *(Cancer Epidemiology, Biomarkers & Prevention 2007; 16(7) – published online ahead of print 10 July 2007)*.

Breast cancer usually comes to light as a painless lump in the breast, but sometimes the lump can be painful to the touch, or there may be breast pain without any obvious lump. If you find a lump in your breast, see your doctor straight away to get it checked out, but don't immediately assume it must be cancer, since around 85 per cent of breast lumps are benign.

Exercise found to lower risk of premenopausal breast cancer

One-fourth of all breast cancers are diagnosed in women before menopause. While numerous studies have shown that physical activity reduces the risk of postmenopausal breast cancer, there is a lack of research into the effects of exercise on premenopausal breast cancer. Now, new research has revealed that girls and young women who exercise regularly between the ages of 12 and 35 have a substantially lower risk of breast cancer before menopause compared to those who are less active.

In the largest and most detailed analysis to date of the effects of exercise on premenopausal breast cancer, the study of nearly 65,000 women found that those who were physically active had a 23 per cent lower risk of breast cancer before menopause. In particular, high levels of physical activity from ages 12 to 22 contributed most strongly to the lower breast cancer risk.

The study was conducted by US researchers at Washington University School of Medicine in St. Louis and Harvard University in Boston.

Commenting on the findings, lead researcher Dr Graham Colditz said: "We don't have a lot of prevention strategies for premenopausal breast cancer, but our findings clearly show that physical activity during adolescence and young adulthood can pay off in the long run by reducing a woman's risk of early breast cancer. This is just one more reason to encourage young girls and women to exercise regularly."

The researchers examined data on a subset of women enrolled in the Nurses' Health Study II, a prospective study of registered nurses ages 24 to 42. These 64,777 women had filled out detailed annual questionnaires about their levels of physical activity from age 12 on. After six years of follow-up, 550 women had been diagnosed with breast cancer.

The researchers found the age-adjusted incidence rates for invasive breast cancer dropped from 194 cases per 100,000 person-years in the least active women to 136 cases in the most active. The levels of physical activity reported by the most active women were the equivalent of running 3.25 hours a week or walking 13 hours a week.

The benefit of exercise was not linked to a particular sport or intensity but related to total activity. "You don't have to be a marathon runner to get the risk-reducing benefits of exercise," Colditz said.

One leading theory to explain the lower risk of breast cancer among active young women is that exercise reduces their exposure to oestrogens. Numerous studies have shown that the more oestrogen a woman is exposed to, the greater her risk for breast cancer. Thus, women who begin menstruating later or enter menopause early have a lower risk of breast cancer. And young women who are physically active are more likely to start their periods later and less likely to have regular cycles when they begin their periods.

Testing for breast cancer – what you need to know:

Breast self-examination:
An effective way to detect breast cancer?

Breast self-examinations may be of limited benefit, according to a study *(Canad. Assoc. Med. J. 164: 1837-46, 2001)*. After analysing the results of several well-controlled trials, the authors concluded that women who carried out this procedure regularly, were at no less risk of dying from breast cancer than women who never examined their breasts.

The *Journal of the National Cancer Institute* published a study which also backed this finding up *(Journal of the National Cancer Institute Oct. 2002; 94(19): 1,445-1,457)*. Researchers studied 266,000 women for 10 years. Half of them were carefully trained and instructed to perform periodic breast examinations and the other half did nothing. At the end of the 10 years, there was no difference between the breast cancer death rates of the two groups.

It's important to bear in mind that almost all breasts are lumpy. They are lumpy because they contain mammary glands that are necessary for milk production. To most people (including most doctors), it is very difficult to distinguish between a lump of mammary gland and a lump of cancer. Yes, it is true that cancer is usually harder than normal glandular tissue, but if there is any fibrous tissue present, it is impossible to distinguish between cancer and, well, not cancer.

This creates all sorts of problems. Women with lumpy breasts are kept in a constant state of anxiety, discovering new lumps, rushing to the doctor, waiting for the biopsy report, wondering 'How much time do I have left? Has it gone to my brain, my bones?' This tragic drama is repeated hundreds of times every week in communities all over the world. Millions of pounds are wasted annually because of women being advised to do an examination they are not qualified to do and, in fact, neither are most doctors.

Unless there is something obvious that needs medical attention, such as bleeding from a nipple or breast pain, try not to panic. In addition, pain in a breast is usually caused by an inflammatory condition (mastitis) or fibrocystic disease. However, it is important that you still get it checked. It's a good idea to get to know what's normal for your breasts in terms of look and texture, so you can spot any changes and get them checked as soon as possible.

Mammograms – an outdated and painful procedure

Once a woman reaches the age of 50, she may start considering taking part in a breast-screening programme. In the UK, this means having a mammogram every three years up to the age of 70.

Women who go to a radiology clinic for their first mammogram are often surprised to find that their breasts must be squeezed between two flat surfaces so the tissue will be sparse enough to allow tumours to be revealed. And you can be certain that it's not a tender squeeze.

To call this uncomfortable is a nice way of saying extremely painful.

But it's also dangerous. The compression required for mammograms can actually break down cancer tissue and rupture small blood vessels that support the cancer, causing it to spread.

This is known as the compression contradiction, and here's what US physician Dr William Campbell Douglass II, has to say about it: "I find it maddeningly contradictory that medical students are taught to examine breasts gently to keep any possible cancer from spreading, yet radiologists are allowed to manhandle them for a mammogram."

When Dr. Douglass says manhandle, that's a nice way of saying squashed flat.

Four common mammography myths...

1. Mammograms are safe. In fact, they're not. As already mentioned, compression of the breast may prompt cancer to spread. And then there's the radiation: A mammogram delivers about 1,000 times more radiation than a chest X-ray and carries a risk of cardiovascular damage.

2. Mammograms catch cancer at an early stage. They don't. In fact, if a tumour is large enough to be detected by a mammogram it's most likely already in an advanced state. Only advanced tumours can be detected.

3. Mammograms save lives. They don't. While there are those who attribute successful cancer treatment to mammogram detection, several studies show that breast cancer mortality is statistically the same among women who have had mammograms and those who haven't. Another study showed that annual mammography screening for women in their 40s, had no effect on a women's risk of dying from breast cancer *(Ann. Int. Med. 137: 305-12, 2002).*

4. Mammograms are the most dependable breast cancer screening method. They're not. There are several safer methods of breast cancer screening that are just as dependable or more dependable than mammography.

Genetics no longer thought to play a big role...

There is growing evidence to suggest that a family history of breast cancer does not play such a big role, as was previously thought to be the case, as an indicator of whether a woman is more likely to develop the disease. Researchers at the Imperial Cancer Research Fund's Cancer Epidemiology Unit, Oxford, in the UK, say that most women with a family history of breast cancer will never develop the disease. Conversely, women who do have breast cancer don't have a close relative with the disease.

However, you should be more wary if you have:

- A relative who was diagnosed under the age of 40
- A close relative with cancer in both breasts
- A male relative with breast cancer
- Two close relatives on the same side of the family diagnosed with breast cancer under 60 or with ovarian cancer
- Three close relatives diagnosed with breast or ovarian cancer at any age

Breast cancer gene clue discovery

Five genetic clues to why some women have a family history of breast cancer have recently been identified by UK researchers. It brings to 18 the number of common genetic variations linked to a small increased risk of breast cancer – they are thought to account for

---

around 8 per cent of inherited cases of breast cancer.

The 18 genetic changes linked to breast cancer are not currently tested for. The Cambridge University-led research, published in Nature Genetics, could see targeted screening and treatment of women more likely to get breast cancer.

In the largest project of its kind and funded by Cancer Research UK, the researchers scanned the entire genetic code of around 4,000 British patients with a family history of breast cancer. They then studied the DNA of another 24,000 women, with and without breast cancer.

The researchers found five 'spots' on the human genome linked to a family history of breast cancer. Another 13 have already been located. Scientists also know about two high risk genes which are more likely to be defective in someone with breast cancer, known as BRCA1 and BRCA2.

Dr Caroline Hacker, policy manager at Breakthrough Breast Cancer, said: "This could lead to new genetic tests which may help identify women who have an increased risk of breast cancer due to inherited faults in genes. Hereditary breast cancer is rare and only around one in 20 of all breast cancers are due to inherited faults in breast cancer genes.

"Although there isn't anything we can do about the genes we inherit, we do know that you can reduce your risk of breast cancer by maintaining a healthy weight, limiting alcohol consumption and exercising regularly."

At present women with a genetic predisposition to breast cancer or a family history of the disease are offered mammography screening, as are those over the age of 50. If a woman is younger than 50 and falls within any of the former two categories, she may begin screening from the age of 30.

The mainstream mantra that all older women should receive a yearly mammogram is so pervasive that many women don't even realize that there are potential hazards to mammography.

A study carried out in Canada concluded that mammography may do more harm than good overall, due to the high number of false positive results (that is, a diagnosis of possible cancer where none exists) *(Lancet 346:29-32, 1995).*

The researchers discovered that only one in every 14 women with a positive result actually had breast cancer, leading to many unnecessary and traumatic surgical operations. Researchers have also found that breast cancer screening isn't a foolproof way of spotting the disease – it fails to detect up to 10-15 per cent of tumours.

A damning report from the Cochrane Collaboration – an independent and prestigious international research organization – revealed that women are being seriously misled by health officials in the way that facts about mammograms are presented *(Cochrane Database System Review. 2009; 4: CD001877; doi: 10.100).*

According to the Cochrane report, health officials are dramatically downplaying the risks of mammography X-rays while overstating the benefits. The report also questions the prevailing view that mammograms save lives and says that this is based on shoddy and biased science.

A different set of facts

The report also found:

• Mammography can save one in 2,000 women screened, or half the official number that is so often quoted by doctors in the UK. This contradicts the statistics offered by Cancer Research UK, which estimates that mammograms can detect seven cancers in every 1,000 women screened.

- Mammograms are carcinogenic because they use X-ray technology. It's estimated that mammograms can cause breast cancer in one out of every 25,000 women screened. This suggests that the procedure can trigger 80 new cases of breast cancer in the UK and around 1,480 new cases in the US, every year.

- A study which tracked 2,400 women aged 40-69 years showed that the rate of false positives increases with the number of times a woman is screened. By the time that a woman has had 10 treatments, the rate of false positives for her could be as high as 64 per cent.

- Screenings can also produce false negatives. In other words, they can fail to detect cancer that is present. Overall, mammograms miss around 20 per cent of cancers in the breast.

The Cochrane researchers concluded that there is no evidence that suggests mammograms are safe, reliable, effective and save lives.

These controversial findings are based on seven studies involving 600,000 women and were judged to be unbiased and truly scientific by the researchers.

Fortunately, there are less invasive and safer alternatives to mammograms, like thermographs... although only a small number of private health clinics currently offer this service in the UK. Perhaps the time has come for this technology to be further developed and embraced as part of a solution to a disease which is a growing health concern for all women.

Thermography: A safe and very effective alternative to mammograms

In an ideal world breast cancer should be detected at its very early stages, before the tumour has grown to a sufficient size. Unfortunately, for the tumour to be detected by a mammogram or physical examination it must've grown for several years, and achieved more than 25 doublings of the malignant cell colony. You guessed it: By the time you get a warning from your mammogram the tumour may already be at a growth-stage where it is too difficult and too late to treat.

So what are the alternatives to this invasive, painful, ineffective and unsafe procedure?

Enter thermography...

Many doctors recognise that inflammation is a precursor to numerous diseases such as cancer, arthritis, heart disease, strokes, diabetes, and high blood pressure. Early detection of inflammation may help you prevent many serious health conditions. You can reduce inflammation with dietary changes, nutritional supplements, antioxidants, detoxification, stress reduction, and more. This is where thermal imaging or thermography comes in to the picture...

This tool creates a digital map of your body that illustrates heat patterns. This may detect some condition or abnormality. It uses an infrared camera that scans and measures your body surface temperature, presenting the information as a digitized image, called a thermograph. These thermal images are analyzed for abnormalities that may be signs of disease in your body. Additionally, since your body is thermally symmetrical if normal, thermal asymmetries can indicate problems.

Benefits, benefits, benefits

Thermograms will be of particular interest to women but men will also find benefit from this tool, as it not only specialises in breast imaging but also excels in early-stage disease detection. For example:

- **Arthritis:** Thermography not only helps detect early signs of arthritis but can also differentiate between osteoarthritis and more severe forms like rheumatoid. Effective early treatment strategies can then be implemented, before you experience further degeneration.

- **Heart Disease:** Screenings can assess heart function and detect inflammation in the carotid arteries (which may be a precursor to stroke and blood clots). Earlier detection of a heart problem may save your life.

- **Neck and Back Pain:** Thermal pain patterns 'light up' white and red hot on a scan. You can get relief faster and begin restorative care that targets the affected area more precisely.

- **Dental Issues:** A thermal scan will indicate temporomandibular joint (TMJ), gum disease, or an infected tooth, as white or red hot.

- **Sinus Issues and Headaches:** Significant heat in your forehead or sinus region revealed on a thermal scan is an indicator that these systems in your body are not functioning properly.

- **Immune Dysfunction, Fibromyalgia and Chronic Fatigue:** The immune system correlates to the T1 and T2 areas of your spine – high levels of heat in that region can indicate immune dysfunction. On the other hand, chronic fatigue, fibromyalgia, and aching joints are just a few complaints that correlate to cool patterns seen at this area.

- **Carpal Tunnel Syndrome (CTS):** This condition is often misdiagnosed. For instance, you may think you have CTS, yet the scan shows your neck is referring pain from a different affected area. This will help you get the most appropriate treatment.

- **Digestive Disorders:** Irritable bowel syndrome, diverticulitis and Crohn's disease are often visible with thermography. If you're able to address these conditions early on, you'll find that health restoration is much more likely.

- **Other Conditions:** Including bursitis, herniated discs, ligament or muscle tear, lupus, nerve problems, whiplash, stroke screening, cancer, and many, many others.

Back to the ladies

Mammograms look at anatomical changes in the breast, as they detect masses or lumps in the breast tissue. On the other hand, thermograms look at vascular changes in the breast, as they detect blood flow patterns, inflammation and asymmetries.

Thermography can detect irregular patterns in the breast, conditions that occur before a noticeable lump is formed. In some cases, such as inflammatory cancer, there are no lumps to be detected by self-examination or mammogram. That's why adding thermography to your annual health routine can help with early detection. You'll increase your chances of detecting breast cancer in its earliest stages.

Unlike most diagnostic tests, thermal imaging is not painful, is non-invasive and quick – your multi-image examinations usually take less than 15 minutes. Plus, it makes no contact with your body – no compression (such as what you experience with mammograms) and it emits absolutely NO radiation.

So, no radiation, no squashing, no mashing and bruising. Early detection, quicker diagnoses and prevention and a healthier happier you.

Breast Cancer Detection System (BCDS) is a method that's completely non-invasive and radiation-free. And, best of all, like thermography it involves no squashing.

BCDS technology is based on the discovery that electricity passes through cancerous tissue differently than it passes through normal tissue. A BCDS device consists of several strips containing electronic sensors that are laid over the breast in a spoke-like pattern. Very low electrical currents are transmitted into the breast without causing any pain to the patient. Diagnosis is made with computer analysis.

An American company called Z-tech is now conducting the final stage of clinical trials with an 18-month test of BCDS at 16 medical centres in the US, Canada and Europe.

What if an abnormality is found following screening?

Doctors may take a sample of tissue using a needle. This is then analysed to assess whether malignant cells are present and confirm the diagnosis of cancer.

The cells may be tested to see if they carry certain receptors, which may influence the treatments offered. If they carry hormone receptors, it suggests they're sensitive to female sex hormones and hormone therapies are likely to be used in their treatment. Cells carrying the HER2 receptor may respond to the drug trastuzumab (Herceptin), which may be used in the treatment of some HER2 positive cancers.

All patients suspected of having breast cancer must be seen by a hospital specialist within two weeks of an urgent referral by their GP. Some hospitals run 'one-stop shops' for rapid assessment of breast lumps where all the examinations can be done on the spot, often with the results available on the same day.

What to expect if your doctor diagnoses breast cancer

Once a diagnosis of breast cancer is confirmed, the exact treatment used, how soon it's given and how long it takes all depends on several factors, including:

- The stage of the tumour (how far it has spread) and whether there is secondary cancer
- The receptor status of the breast cancer
- Fitness and wellbeing

- If you've had the menopause
- Your own wishes on the treatments you may receive

The mainstay of conventional breast cancer treatment is surgery. If the tumour is caught early, only it and the immediate surrounding tissue needs to be removed, in a process called lumpectomy, which is usually accompanied by radiotherapy. In more advanced cases a mastectomy (removal of the whole breast) is performed.

Chemotherapy or hormone-blocking drugs (such as tamoxifen) may accompany either procedure. Tamoxifen is also recommended by some doctors as a preventive medication.

Tamoxifen works by blocking the female hormone oestrogen. This hormone acts as a chemical messenger throughout the body including the skin, gut, brain and breasts, to promote healthy cell growth.

But oestrogen's role can have a devastating impact in the presence of breast cancer cells. Many breast tumours are hormone-responsive – when exposed to oestrogen the cancer cells may begin to multiply at an alarming rate.

Tamoxifen latches on to oestrogen 'receptor' sites in both healthy and cancerous breast cells, thereby preventing the exposure of the cells to oestrogen. In this way, it helps stop the proliferation of cancer cells.

But research has shown that tamoxifen can 'turn' on its user – sometimes in a matter of months or sometimes after years of usage. In these cases the tumour cells themselves become tamoxifen-resistant and the drug stops working, allowing cancer cells to spread. Tamoxifen can cause unpleasant side effects such as nausea, hot flushes, vaginal discharge, vaginal bleeding and, if taken for a long period, eye damage. It has also been linked with an increase of cancer of the womb, stroke and potentially fatal blood clots.

A drug called Herceptin is also available. It's been designed to be used along with chemotherapy and/or radiation to treat a type of breast cancer called HER2. About one in four breast cancers are HER2 positive. However, despite its ability to reduce the expression of HER2, it has been linked to an increased risk of heart problems.

Surgery carries the risk of post-operative infection, while chemotherapy and radiotherapy have many unpleasant side effects and may cause permanent damage for a few per cent of patients.

How to combat anaemia caused by radiation therapy

When breast cancer is treated with radiation, the body is assaulted twice: once by the disease and once by the therapy. A new study shows how women fighting breast cancer can easily and safely alleviate some of the harshest effects of radiation therapy: including anaemia.

Red blood cells deliver oxygen from the lungs to tissues throughout the body. Anaemia occurs when the red blood cell count becomes depleted, resulting in fatigue, weakness, and hair loss in extreme cases. The two primary causes of anaemia are: 1) iron deficiency (often triggered by menstruation or internal bleeding), and 2) deficiency of two key vitamins: folate and vitamin B12. Radiation therapy also causes anaemia.

US researchers at the University of Michigan evaluated 20 women receiving radiation for breast cancer who participated in an exercise intervention study:

- Half the women were randomly assigned to a group that took aerobic exercise three to five days each week by walking for 20 to 45 minutes.

- The other women participated in stretching exercises three to five days each week.

- Blood was drawn from each subject before and after the seven-week study period.

- Results showed that peak aerobic capacity (measured with oxygen uptake analysis) increased by more than six per cent in the walking group, but decreased by more than four per cent in the stretching group.

- Red blood cell count increased significantly in the walking group, but decreased in the stretching group.

- Haemoglobin (a red blood cell protein that helps transfer oxygen from the lungs to the body) increased significantly in the walking group, but decreased in the stretching group.

- Researchers noted that the walking exercise in this study was only of moderate intensity, but still provided a "safe, economical method" to improve fitness and maintain healthy red blood cell status.

Anaemia is often referred to as 'iron poor blood'. But care should be taken when treating anaemia with iron supplements.

US physician and *HSI* panellist Dr Allan Spreen cautions that supplemental iron may create problems in high doses: "The RDA of iron is far too high. Plus, even if you were proven to have anaemia I wouldn't treat it with inorganic iron. The mineral is too reactive in the body when it is not insulated from the system by being encased within the haem structure of haemoglobin. Free radical formation from free iron is just too much of a threat."

Dietary sources of haem iron come exclusively from red meat, fish, pork, and poultry, with beef liver and chicken liver having the highest amounts of iron. An additional intake of vitamin C can also help the body absorb iron.

Supplements of folic acid and vitamin B12 may also help address anaemia. The recommended daily allowance (RDA) for folate is 400mcg, but Dr Spreen recommends folic acid supplementation of 1,600mcg per day, noting, "folate isn't effective in low doses except in a limited percentage of cases."

Along with folate, Dr Spreen recommends 1,000mcg of B12 per day in sublingual form (dissolved under the tongue). Dr Spreen suggests that to get the most out of folic acid, add 100mg per day of B6, as well as 400-500mg of magnesium per day to make the B6 more effective.

Talk with your doctor or a health care professional before including these supplements in your daily regimen.

Maximise your chances of beating breast cancer with these natural remedies

Natural remedies can play an important role in the fight against breast cancer when used, with your doctor's prior approval, alongside conventional treatments. There is evidence that some are able to prevent the disease and even help combat existing cases from spreading (metastasising) to other organs.

It is extremely important that cancer patients inform their doctor before self-medicating with any of the supplements listed, and their progress should be carefully monitored by their doctor.

- **Antioxidants may help guard against the disease**. Antioxidants eliminate reactive molecules called free radicals, which may cause cancer to develop by damaging the DNA inside cells. The major dietary antioxidants are vitamins C, E and A, selenium and the carotenes. Good protective daily dosages would be 2g vitamin C; 400 IU vitamin E; 15,000 IU vitamin A (7,500 IU max in pregnancy); 200mcg selenium and 10,000 IU beta-carotene.

A new study has shown that women with breast cancer have significantly lower levels of antioxidants in their blood than healthy women, with beta-carotene appearing to be especially low *(J. Nutr. 132: 303-6, 2002)*. Co-enzyme Q10 (CoQ10) is a powerful antioxidant that also boosts your immune system's natural defences against cancer.

In a Danish study, researchers gave 390mg of CoQ10 a day to a group of women with breast cancer that was already spreading to other parts of their bodies. After several months, the researchers found that the cancer went into remission for four of the women. In one woman the cancer completely disappeared after 11 months *(Biochem. Biophys. Res. Comm. 212: 172-7, 1995)*. As part of a preventive programme of antioxidants, 60mg a day is recommended.

- **How protection from breast cancer could be found from an unlikely source**

Although free radicals are normally damaging to the body, new research on a compound called artemisinin, isolated from the herb sweet wormwood *(Artemisia annua)* shows that in certain circumstances they can be targeted specifically to kill cancerous cells *(Life Sciences 70: 49-56, 2001)*.

Breast cancer cells contain higher amounts of iron than healthy breast cells and when artemisinin combines with iron, free radicals are generated causing the cells to die. Although more research in this area is needed, laboratory studies conducted so far have shown that artemisinin killed about 30 per cent of breast cancer cells. And when combined with transferrin (a molecule that increases the uptake of iron by cells), a staggering 98 per cent of cancerous cells were destroyed. Normal breast cells were only minimally affected, suggesting that the artemisinin and transferrin combination could promise a safe, new treatment for breast cancer.

- **Taking fish oil supplements can lower your risk of breast cancer by up to 32%**

Researchers have found that taking fish oil supplements on a regular basis could help protect against breast cancer *(the American Association for Cancer Research journal Cancer Epidemiology, Biomarkers & Prevention, published online on 8 July 2010)*. Fish oil contains high amounts of eicosapentaenoic acid (EPA) and docosahexaenoic acid (DHA) – omega-3 fatty acids that are frequently lacking in modern diets.

The current study included 35,016 postmenopausal women who were members of the VITamins And Lifestyle (VITAL) Cohort. Questionnaires completed from 2000 to 2002 provided information concerning the frequency and duration of use of non-vitamin, non-mineral supplements including fish oil supplements, and those that target menopausal symptoms, such as black cohosh.

At the six year follow-up, 880 cases of breast cancer were diagnosed among the participants. Women who had reported regular use of fish oil supplements had a 32 per cent lower risk of invasive ductal breast cancer, the most common form of the disease, compared to non-users. Other supplements did not appear to effect breast cancer risk. This study is the first to reveal an association between supplementing with fish oil and a decrease in breast cancer risk.

- **Black cohosh can reduce your risk of breast cancer by over 60%**

Black cohosh root extract is widely used as an alternative to hormone replacement therapy (HRT), to reduce menopause symptoms. Recently, US scientists at the University of Pennsylvania Medical School who carried out a case control study on almost 2,500 women, found that those who took supplements of black cohosh had an astounding 61 per cent reduction in their breast cancer risk *(Int J Cancer 2007; 120(7): 1523-1528)*.

Black cohosh contains two kinds of biologically active compounds, called triterpene glycosides and cinnamic acid esters. Both of these plant chemicals have been shown in laboratory experiments to reduce the growth of human breast cancer cells and to increase the rate at which these cells die off *(Biol Pharmaceut Bull 2004; 27(12): 1970).*

The recommended daily dosage is 100mg to 250mg of black cohosh root extract, standardised to contain 2.5 per cent triterpene glycosides. Black cohosh should not be taken during pregnancy.

- **Vitamins and calcium supplements can lower breast cancer risk**

Vitamins and calcium supplements can significantly reduce the risk of breast cancer – even when they're taken at the standard daily dose. Vitamin supplements reduce the risk by around 30 per cent, and calcium supplements by 40 per cent.

However, the researchers were quick to point out that the supplements must be taken every day over an extended period of time in order to produce these beneficial effects.

Commenting on the findings, Dr Jaime Matta, one of the researchers from the Ponce School of Medicine in Puerto Rico, said: "It is not an immediate effect. You don't take a vitamin today and your breast cancer risk is reduced tomorrow" *(Presentation at the American Association for Cancer Research 101st Annual Meeting, April 17-21, 2010, Washington, DC).*

- **Vitamin D helps block the growth of blood vessels that feed breast cancer cells**

Upping your vitamin D intake may also help to ward off breast cancer. A study at Birmingham University and St George's Hospital, London, discovered that breast tissue contains an enzyme that converts vitamin D to its active form, calcitriol, which is a potent anti-cancer agent *(J Nutr 2006: 136: 887-892)*. Levels of the enzyme were elevated in breast tumours – suggesting that calcitriol is produced as a natural defence mechanism to combat the spread of cancer.

Other research has shown that calcitriol not only inhibits breast cancer cells from multiplying, it also makes those cells grow and die more like natural cells. What's more, vitamin D inhibits the growth of blood vessels that feed the cancerous tumour – a process called anti-angiogenesis *(Braz J Med Biol Res 2002; 35(1): 1-9)*.

According to a population study published earlier this year, vitamin D exposure through diet, supplements and sunshine is directly related to a reduced risk of breast cancer *(Cancer Epidemiol Biomarkers Prev 2007; 16(3): 422–9)*. Vitamin D acts as a hormone in the body and too much of it can lead to calcium being deposited in the arteries, so it's important not to overdose on it. Take no more than 10mcg to 30mcg daily (400 IU to 1,200 IU).

Ginseng could improve breast cancer patients' quality of life

QOL is an acronym for quality of life. When QOL is good, we may not give it much thought on a day-to-day basis. But when life is challenged with a serious health crisis, QOL often becomes a moment-to-moment issue.

For women who are diagnosed with breast cancer, quality of life and even survival chances may improve with the use of a herbal treatment with a history that stretches back many centuries.

Two intriguing comments were made by a researcher at the conclusion of a study that tracked ginseng use among breast cancer patients:

• When patients used ginseng prior to diagnosis, they tended to have higher survival.

- Ginseng use after cancer diagnosis was related to improved quality of life.

Both of those observations were made by Dr Xiao-Ou Shu, Ph.D., of the Vanderbilt-Ingram Cancer Center at Vanderbilt University Medical Center a facility that focuses on an interdisciplinary approach to cancer care, treatment and prevention.

A Vanderbilt press release (the source of Dr Shu's comments) notes that there are two primary classes of ginseng: red and white. White ginseng root is naturally dried and is reputed to promote general good health over a long period. Red ginseng gets its colour from a drying process that increases potency. This variety is used by some herbalists to aid disease recovery.

Benefits of cumulative use

Shu's team (which included a representative from the Shanghai Cancer Institute) recruited more than 1,450 subjects who joined the Shanghai Breast Cancer Study between 1996 and 1998. Information on the subjects' ginseng use before and after breast cancer diagnosis was gathered through the end of 2002.

Nearly 30 per cent of the subjects were regular ginseng users before their cancer diagnosis. Researchers found that these subjects had a significantly reduced risk of death compared to subjects who never used ginseng. Meanwhile, ginseng use after diagnosis was associated with higher QOL scores, especially in the areas of psychological and social well-being. The authors add: "QOL improved as cumulative ginseng use increased."

Each of the subjects also underwent some form of conventional cancer treatments, such as chemotherapy, radiation therapy and surgery.

The Vanderbilt press release notes that the study was limited in that subjects didn't specify what ginseng varieties they used or how the ginseng was prepared. In addition, subjects were not asked about other alternative therapies they might have been using at the same time.

For now, Dr Shu continues to collect data on subjects in the Shanghai group and also from another breast cancer study with about 4,000 subjects. She hopes to mount a placebo-controlled trial in the near future.

• Indole-3-carbinol: A natural breakthrough in the fight against breast cancer

For most women one of their greatest fears in life is developing breast cancer. In recent years much hope has been pinned on the drug tamoxifen which has been used to both treat and prevent breast cancer.

Tamoxifen has undoubtedly done much to help reduce the death rate and prevent recurrence of the disease. However, its success has been overshadowed by a number of harmful side effects associated with its use. Scientists are constantly looking for a safer alternative to tamoxifen, to use instead of, or as an adjunct to chemotherapy.

Now a natural chemical called indole-3-carbinol is provoking much interest from both mainstream and alternative medicine. To fully understand how indole-3-carbinol works, it is important to first explore the role of tamoxifen in fighting breast cancer.

Tamoxifen: the anti-cancer drug linked with harmful side-effects

As mentioned on page 40, tamoxifen works by blocking the female hormone oestrogen. This hormone acts as a chemical messenger throughout the body including the skin, gut, brain and breasts, to promote healthy cell growth.

But oestrogen's role can have a devastating impact in the presence of breast cancer cells. Many breast tumours are hormone-responsive – when exposed to oestrogen the cancer cells may begin to multiply at an alarming rate.

Tamoxifen latches on to oestrogen 'receptor' sites in both healthy and cancerous breast cells, thereby preventing the exposure of the cells to oestrogen. In this way, it helps stop the proliferation of cancer cells.

But research has shown that tamoxifen can 'turn' on its user – sometimes in a matter of months or sometimes after years of usage. In these cases the tumour cells themselves become tamoxifen-resistant and the drug stops working, allowing cancer cells to spread. It can cause unpleasant side effects such as nausea, hot flushes, vaginal discharge, vaginal bleeding and, if taken for a long period, eye damage. The drug has also been linked with an increase of cancer of the womb, stroke and potentially fatal blood clots.

Indole-3-carbinol makes oestrogen a weaker and less destructive force

Indole-3-carbinol provides a natural alternative treatment in the management of breast cancer. It helps prevent the growth of cancer cells and can even destroy existing ones. This chemical occurs naturally in cruciferous vegetables – in which four petal flowers resemble a cross – such as broccoli, kale and Brussels sprouts. It has long been recognised as a potent substance and has been the subject of intense research in relation to cancer.

In 1991, researchers at the Institute for Hormone Research in New York, announced that by using indole-3-carbinol they had been able to convert the stronger form of oestrogen (known as oestradiol) into a weaker form (2-hydroxyestrone), by up to 50 per cent in 12 healthy people *(Nutr Cancer. 1991;16(1): 59-66)*. 2-hydroxyestrone is considered to be a more 'desirable' form of oestrogen in the body, as it effectively blocks the strong 'grow' signals oestradiol sends to cancer cells.

116

Then in 1997, researchers at the Strang Cancer Research Laboratory in New York, found that when indole-3-carbinol changes oestradiol into the weaker form, it stops human cancer cells from growing by up to 61 per cent and provokes the cells into self-destructing *(J. Cell Biochem Supplement 1997. 28-29: 111-6).*

Subsequent studies done at Berkeley in California show that indole-3-carbinol inhibits a certain type of human breast cancer cell from growing by as much as 90 per cent in laboratory experiments *(Cancer Research. 1999; 59; 1244-1251).* Leonard Bjeldanes, co-author of the study, says: "Indole-3-carbinol hits the cancer from a different angle than other anti-cancer drugs which makes it a very powerful and interesting chemical. What is also exciting, is that indole-3-carbinol has low toxicity but is a very effective agent against mammary tumours."

Combined with tamoxifen it can reduce the spread of cancer cells by 95 per cent!

Even more astonishingly, when indole-3-carbinol was combined with tamoxifen it appeared to limit the drug's potentially harmful side effects while amplifying its anti-oestrogen properties.

Berkeley researchers injected three groups of human breast cancer cells – one with indole-3-carbinol, one with tamoxifen, and one with the two substances combined. The cells injected with tamoxifen alone showed a 60 per cent inhibition of cancer cells, while the cells injected with indole-3-carbinol showed a 90 per cent inhibition. But the combination of the two worked even better – resulting in a staggering 95 per cent inhibition *(Cancer Research. 1999; 59; 1244-1251).*

This means that women who need to take tamoxifen can combine it with indole-3-carbinol to maximise its effects. In some cases they may be able to reduce their dosage, and in doing so decrease the likelihood of resistance to the drug. But please: Do not attempt to reduce the dose of your cancer drugs without consulting your doctor first.

Could eating more broccoli protect you from breast cancer?

Unfortunately, simply increasing your intake of broccoli and cabbage to boost your levels of indole-3-carbinol is not enough. You should include plenty of these healthful vegetables in your diet of course. But in order to consume enough cruciferous vegetables to have a positive effect, you would need to eat at least a pound or more of cabbage or cauliflower daily! However, the good news is that indole-3-carbinol is now available in supplement form.

Dosage instructions: The recommended dose is between one and four capsules daily, depending on your weight (6-7mg per kg of weight per day).

Further investigation of indole-3-carbinol has shown that it is more effective when taken in conjunction with vitamin C. The combination produces fat-soluble ascorbigen, which is an effective anti-carcinogen *(Preobrazhenskaya et al Food Chemistry. 1993; 48: 48-52)*.

Warning: If you are suffering from breast cancer (particularly if you are taking tamoxifen) please consult your doctor before taking indole-3-carbinol. Pregnant women should not take indole-3-carbinol.

Study shows how support groups improve the survival rates of breast cancer patients

Here's an effective cancer-fighter with a guarantee of no adverse side effects: talk.

Breast cancer sufferers had better survival rates when they participated in weekly sessions with other cancer survivors and a clinical psychologist.

Researchers at the Comprehensive Cancer Center at Ohio State University, in the US, recruited more than 220 women who had received surgery to address breast cancer *("Intervention Boosts Breast Cancer Survival" Ivanhoe Newswire, 11/19/08, ivanhoe.com)*. Half participated in the weekly sessions for four months (sessions were conducted monthly for an additional eight months), and half did not. Patients in the intervention group were also given tips to improve health behaviours and reduce stress.

The Ohio State team followed up to assess the health of all the subjects about a decade later:

- Patients who participated in the intervention group and later died lived for an average of 6.1 years

- Patients who didn't participate in the intervention group and later died lived for an average of 4.8 years

- Patients in the intervention group were also less likely to die of other cancers or heart disease

See the Helpful Organisations section on page 319 for contact details of cancer support groups.

• Breast-Mate™ – this ground-breaking mushroom remedy helps stop breast cancer in its tracks

Traditional Asian medicine is often way ahead of Western medicine... and that's becoming glaringly obvious in the fight against cancer. Now, one ancient remedy has been married with today's technology, creating a formula so powerful that it is able to target breast cancer cells before they grow and multiply – helping to stop the disease in its tracks.

Japanese doctors have seen remarkable results: In one breast cancer patient, doctors saw a ping pong ball-sized tumour disappear after just two months of treatment with phellinus linteus (PL) – a medicinal mushroom extract (called meshima in Japan).

When the Maitake Products Inc (MPI) – a US-based company which harnesses the medicinal powers of mushrooms, like maitake, in its wide range of nutritional supplements – research and development team learned about PL they knew it would become the centerpiece of their new formula Breast-Mate.™

Breast-Mate™ was specifically formulated to support healthy breast cells – but it appears to do much more than that.

Building on Dr Sliva's Success

MPI became interested in PL after learning about the work of a scientist called Dr Daniel Sliva. In the course of his 10-year research on medicinal mushrooms, Dr Sliva and his team found undeniable evidence in the lab that an extract of PL has a four-fold anti-breast-cancer effect (*British Journal of Cancer, 2008*):

1. It inhibits cell adhesion, meaning it keeps breast cancer cells from joining together to form tumours.
2. It restricts cell migration, so breast cancer cells can't move to other areas of the body (known as metastases).
3. It curbs cell invasion, meaning the PL extract doesn't let breast cancer cells take over healthy cells.
4. It suppresses angiogenesis, which is the formation of new blood vessels – something tumours can't live without.

On top of that, the PL extract decreased cancer cell multiplication by up to 78 per cent!

It turns out that Dr Sliva wasn't the only one who'd seen phenomenal anti-cancer effects with PL extract. Back in 1970, a group of Japanese researchers induced sarcoma (cancerous tumours) in mice. PL mushroom extracts caused complete tumour regression in more than half of the mice... and demonstrated inhibition ratios (meaning that tumour growth stopped) over 95 per cent... with absolutely no toxicity *(Chem. Pharm. Bull. 1971)*. In 2009, researchers uncovered yet another key component of PL, called hispolon, that causes apoptosis (cell death) in breast and bladder cancer cells *(Food and Chemical Toxicology 2009)*.

A cultured version of PL was approved as a medicine in 1997 in Korea, and has been used there as medication ever since – sometimes in conjunction with standard chemotherapy, and sometimes as a stand-alone treatment for cancer patients.

Five proven cancer-fighters join the PL fraction

While PL is the key ingredient in the Breast-Mate™ formula, it's not the only ingredient proven to have a powerful impact on breast cancer:

1. Maitake Standardized Extract PSX fraction™. Maitake mushrooms have a long and rich history when it comes to fighting breast cancer. But it turns out that a special extract, the PSX Fraction, can take on breast cancer from another angle entirely.

In 2003, the PSX fraction (different to the maitake extract researchers had been pitting against cancer cells) was found to lower blood sugar better than a prescription drug *(Medicine Update 2002; Molecular and Cellular Biochemistry 2007)*.

You may be wondering what lower blood sugar and increased insulin sensitivity have to do with breast cancer. Dr Cun Zhuang of MPI explains why the PSX fraction was used instead of the proven cancer-fighting D fraction: "It is said that cancer feeds on sugar, and the relationship between high blood sugar and cancer (especially breast cancer) has been discussed more and more these days. Maitake

SX-fraction is a proprietary extract that improves insulin resistance, making it effective for people with Metabolic Syndrome and Type 2 Diabetes *(Lancet Oncology 2005; Cancer Epidemiology, Biomarkers & Prevention (2009); International Journal of Cancer 2006)."*

2. Broccoli extract. As already mentioned, broccoli contains indole 3 carbinol (I3C) – a compound that's been found to be highly beneficial in the fight against breast cancer. In fact, back in 1995, scientists found that I3C could actually prevent breast tumours in rodents *(Annals of the New York Academy of Sciences 1995).*

Then in 1999, researchers found that using I3C in combination with tamoxifen (a common chemotherapy drug used on breast cancer patients) better halted the growth of oestrogen-dependent breast cancer cells (known as MCF-7 cells) than the drug on its own *(Cancer Research 1999).*

It appears that I3C activates a pathway that stops the cycle of human breast cancer cells (specifically, MCF-7 cells) *(Carcinogenesis 2004).* It also produces a substance called DIM (3,3'- diindolylmethane) during digestion, and DIM performs a critical job... it prevents oestrone from turning into its cancer-causing form, 16-hydroxyestrone... stopping cancer cells before they can get started.

3. Green tea extract is well-known for its breast cancer-fighting properties. One study in particular found that women with breast cancer who drank green tea had the least cancer spread... and that women who drank at least five cups a day before their diagnoses were less likely to have their cancer recur *(Japanese Journal of Cancer Research 1998).*

Green tea appears to get its cancer-fighting powers from a component called EGCG (epigallocatechin gallate), which inhibits the growth of cancer cells without doing any damage to healthy cells *(Cancer Letters 1998).* Scientists discovered that EGCG could inhibit breast cancer cells transplanted into mice by up to 99 per cent *(Cancer Letters 1995)*.

In 2007, researchers learned that EGCG along with other polyphenols found in green tea could slow down breast cancer tumour growth, shrink tumours, and set off breast cancer cell death in mice (who'd been injected with human breast cancer cells).

4 & 5. Vitamin D3 and folic acid. As mentioned on page 112, women who get more dietary vitamin D and more exposure to sunlight have been found to have a substantially reduced risk of developing breast cancer. Not only that, but vitamin D also helps prevent tumours from growing.

Studies have shown that a higher intake of folic acid is linked with a decreased risk of breast cancer – a decrease of up to 29 per cent *(Cancer Research. 2001)*. And the benefit is even stronger when women get plenty of 'folate cofactors' like vitamins B6 and B12.

What to take for best results

The recommended dosage for Breast-Mate™ is one to two tablets taken twice a day, or as otherwise recommended by your healthcare practitioner. As always, it's important to consult your doctor prior to using this product, especially if you're taking any medication to lower your blood sugar, as the supplement contains the blood-sugar lowering ingredient Maitake SX-fraction.

Two simple lifestyle changes that can help ward off breast cancer

A study published in the journal *Cancer* reports on two very simple preventative measures, which most of us could easily incorporate into our daily lives, to significantly decrease our risk of a specific type of breast cancer.

The first involves ductal carcinoma in situ (DCIS) – often considered an early marker of breast cancer that's confined to the milk glands or the ducts that carry milk from the glands to the nipple. DCIS is highly curable when diagnosed early. But when not discovered in the formative stages, this condition commonly develops into invasive breast cancer.

A high level of hormones circulating in the body has been associated with an increased risk of breast cancer. Knowing that exercise may reduce the total amount of circulating hormones, researchers at the University of Southern California (USC) launched the first study of how physical activity impacts DCIS.

The USC team began by examining data from a population-based study in Los Angeles County. From that study, more than 550 women diagnosed with DCIS were personally interviewed by the USC researchers. More than 600 women in a cancer-free control group were also interviewed. Subjects ranged in age from 35 to 64 years.

After adjusting for several cancer risk factors, researchers found that women who reported any exercise activity were at 35 per cent lower risk of DCIS than women who could be described as inactive. The lead author of the study, Dr Leslie Bernstein, told Reuters Health News that for invasive disease, "the risk decreased proportionally with increasing level of exercise."

Unfortunately, there was one group that showed no reduction in risk associated with exercise: those women who had a first-degree family history (such as a mother or sister) of DCIS.

The second step involves drinking green tea. In one study, extracts of green tea inhibited breast cancer cells from manufacturing the new blood vessels necessary to promote cancer cell growth. And in another USC population-based study of almost 1,100 women, researchers found that women who drank less than half a cup of green tea daily reduced their breast cancer risk by nearly 30 per cent.

These are two very simple preventive measures – moderate exercise and a small amount of green tea intake – that most of us could easily incorporate into our daily habits to significantly decrease our risk of breast cancer. Other lifestyle risk factors that can be addressed to lower breast cancer risk include smoking, HRT use, excessive alcohol intake, and obesity.

• Increase your chances of beating breast cancer with this ground-breaking new complementary remedy

Protective Breast Formula™ contains a combination of clinically and scientifically studied natural ingredients – including grape seed extract, green tea, turmeric, diindolylmethane (a natural plant chemical from cabbages), maitake mushroom, vitamin D and calcium D-glucarate (a natural body chemical) – that protect breast health in a variety of ways.

Together these ingredients provide important immune system support, promote healthy cell development, act as hormone detoxifiers and help fight cancer-causing free radicals.

Antioxidants in grape seed extract and green tea prevent breast cancer growth

Human cells are constantly exposed to damaging, unstable molecules called free radicals, which have been strongly implicated in causing many diseases, including cancer. Whilst your body is able to produce antioxidants to neutralise these harmful molecules, sometimes it requires extra help.

Grape seed extract is a very powerful antioxidant, several times more effective than vitamin C or vitamin E in quenching free radicals. In animal studies, grape seed extract has been linked to a 50 per cent reduction in breast cancer incidence. When rats were fed a diet containing grape seed extract and then given a chemical known to cause breast cancer, they developed only half the number of tumours as the control group *(J Nutr 2004; 134 (12 Suppl): 3445S-3452S).*

As reported earlier, green tea is another powerful antioxidant, which also has the remarkable ability to cause cancerous cells to die, without affecting normal cells. In laboratory studies involving human breast cancer tissue, a compound present in green tea called epigallocatechin gallate (EGCG) was able to block the multiplication of cancer cells by up to 100 per cent and reduce their viability by up to 78 per cent *(Mol Cancer Ther 2005; 4(1): 81-90).*

An epidemiological study in South-East China, concluded that the regular consumption of green tea has a protective effect against breast cancer *(Carcinogenesis 2007; 28(5): 1074-1078).*

Curcumin – the Indian spice that is able to 'switch off' breast cancer genes

Curcumin, the active ingredient in the Indian spice turmeric, has long been hailed as a powerful antioxidant and anti-inflammatory substance *(Phytother Res 2004; 18(10): 798-804).* Laboratory studies have established that it also works in a variety of different ways to suppress breast cancer. These include counteracting the cancer-promoting effects of the hormone oestrogen, blocking the development of the blood supply that feeds a tumour, and preventing tumours from spreading *(J Cancer 2002; 98(2): 234-40).*

US scientists from the Anderson Cancer Center in Houston, Texas, have found that curcumin blocks the action of a protein called 'nuclear factor Kappa B', which 'switches on' the genes that allow breast cancer to develop and grow. Specifically, curcumin appears to be able to prevent the uncontrolled growth of breast tumour cells, to restore the normal mechanism by which cells die and to prevent cancer spread (metastasis) through the bloodstream and lymphatic system *(Clin Cancer Res 2005; 11: 7490-7498)*.

The incredible anti-cancer compounds in cabbage and broccoli

Breast cancer is a hormone-dependent cancer that is linked to oestrogen, and especially to a 'strong' form of oestrogen called oestradiol. Cruciferous vegetables (members of the cabbage family) contain a plant chemical called indole-3-carbinol (I3C) that has been linked to a reduced risk of cancer *(JAMA 285: 2975-7, 2001)*.

In the gut, I3C is broken down into another substance, diindolylmethane (DIM), which has been found to actively inhibit the growth of breast cancer tumours in rats *(Carcinogenesis 1998; 19(9): 1631-1639)*. In a small pilot study of Californian women with early stage breast cancer, DIM increased the breakdown of oestrogen and oestradiol into harmless and even beneficial compounds *(Nutr Cancer 2004; 50(2): 161-167)*.

Another natural compound that helps to break down oestrogen and cancer-promoting toxins is calcium D-glucarate. This chemical is produced in your body and also in cruciferous plants. When scientists fed rats a diet containing calcium D-glucarate and then exposed them to a breast cancer-causing chemical, the rats developed 70 per cent less tumours than the control group and showed an associated drop in their levels of oestradiol *(Carcinogenesis 1986; 7(9): 1463-1466)*.

How maitake mushrooms and vitamin D boost natural killer cells and starve tumours

Your immune system is your body's first line of defence against cancer. An extract of maitake mushrooms (*Grifola frondosa*) has been found to support the immune system by boosting the activity of 'natural killer' cells, which detect and destroy invading organisms and abnormal body cells *(Biol Pharm Bull 2002; 25(12):1647-1650)*. In a clinical trial, maitake extract not only stimulated natural killer cell activity but also slowed breast cancer progression and prevented the spread (metastasis) of tumours *(J Med Food 2003; 6(4): 371-377)*.

While vitamin D is best known for supporting healthy bones, scientific studies have found that it also encourages healthy breast tissue growth and strengthens the immune system *(J Steroid Biochem Mol Biol 2004; 89-90(1-5): 245-249)*.

In addition, laboratory studies have revealed that the biologically active form of vitamin D, called D3, actually hastens the death of breast cancer cells *(Ann NY Acad Sci 2003; 1010: 437-440)*. Better still, vitamin D also inhibits the growth of blood vessels that feed the cancerous tumour (a process called anti-angiogenesis), literally starving it to death *(Braz J Med Biol Res 2002; 35(1): 1-9)*.

What to take for best results

The recommended dosage for Protective Breast Formula™ is one or two tablets taken twice a day with food. Pregnant or nursing mothers and women taking prescription medication should check with their doctor before using this product.

- ## How a product derived from wheatgerm is outperforming many leading conventional drugs... including tamoxifen

Nancy Henry was diagnosed with breast cancer in May of 2004. Two years and two mastectomies later, the worst was confirmed – the cancer had spread throughout her lungs.

After suffering a series of horrendous side effects from conventional treatments, Nancy's doctor determined that her body was too sensitive for chemotherapy. For the same reason, Nancy decided she would not be taking any more drugs to fight her cancer either.

Even though she was told her life expectancy wouldn't be long if she turned her back on conventional treatments entirely, Nancy decided instead to focus on her quality of life. Because, after all, what use is a prolonged life if it's one of pain and suffering?

And then something amazing happened. Once Nancy changed her focus, turning to a self-designed programme including exercise, visualization, detoxification, supplements, and a stricter approach to her diet, her condition started to gradually improve and her energy levels increased. Avemar – an incredible cancer-fighter derived from wheat germ – is just one part of Nancy's, as she calls it, 'dance with cancer'. However, she believes it could be the most important part.

Her last PET/CAT scan, taken about six months ago, showed that her cancer is classified as 'stable metastatic disease'. Nancy says this is the best you can hope for when you have cancer like hers, where numerous tumours are spread throughout the lungs.

Most of the tumours, while they hadn't gone away, were static. Only six of those many tumours were actually growing, and at a rate far slower than would be expected from even the least aggressive Grade 1 cancer, which is nothing short of astounding.

A cancer fighter that actually boosts your immune system

Who knew that something as simple as wheat germ could hold the key to fighting such a serious disease without the toxic side effects associated with most cancer treatments? Surprisingly enough, someone knew as early as World War I.

Dr Albert Szent-Györgyi, who later went on to win the Nobel Prize for his discovery of vitamin C, was determined to find an alternative to the dangerous mustard gas being used to fight cancer.

When his early research was finally published in the 1960s, it showed that a compound in wheat germ prohibited cancer cells from growing while allowing healthy cells to live normally.

However, instead of following up on his research the scientific community decided they'd rather focus on chemotherapy and radiation treatments that leave the body ravaged – killing cancer cells and healthy cells alike, without discrimination.

Fortunately, in 1989, Dr Maté Hidvégi, a Hungarian biochemist, picked up where Dr Szent-Györgyi left off, eventually patenting a technique of fermenting wheat germ with baker's yeast. This marked the creation of Avemar, which is produced by American BioSciences. Backed up by 100 reports and 20 peer-reviewed publications, Avemar has become a standard therapy for cancer patients in Hungary.

Avemar helps cut off cancer cells' energy supply by interacting with glucose, which normally fuels the spread of tumours. It also keeps cancer cells from repairing themselves by reducing the production of RNA and DNA associated with the rapid reproduction of those cells. Not only does Avemar help kill cancer cells, but it also enhances the immune system by increasing the number and activity of functioning immune-system cells.

More powerful than tamoxifen but without the drug's dangerous side effects

In a study on mice injected with breast cancer tissue, Avemar inhibited the growth of one kind of oestrogen-sensitive breast cancer by 50 per cent, as compared to the conventional breast cancer drug tamoxifen, which inhibited it by 34 per cent.

For another kind of oestrogen-sensitive breast cancer, Avemar had an inhibition rate of 49 per cent. Tamoxifen had a rate of 42 per cent.

Avemar works better than two other commonly used anti-hormone breast cancer drugs as well. Anastrozole (Arimidex) inhibited cancer cell growth by only 25 per cent, and exemestane (Aromasin) fared only slightly better with a rate of 26 per cent.

Against a kind of breast cancer that is not oestrogen-sensitive, Avemar inhibited growth by 52 per cent. The other drugs in the study don't even work against cancers that aren't oestrogen-sensitive.

Although Avemar beat these three popular cancer drugs, the best effects were achieved in combination. The best combination was that of Aromasin and Avemar, which inhibited growth of the breast cancer cells by 60.4 per cent *(Journal of Clinical Oncology, 2007; 25: 18 (June 20 Supplement))*.

About 75 per cent of breast cancers are oestrogen receptor-positive. This means there are a significant number of receptors for the hormone oestrogen on the surface of the breast cancer cells.

When oestrogen in the bloodstream attaches to these receptors, signals are sent to the cell nucleus, telling the cancer cell to grow and divide. When it comes to fighting oestrogen-sensitive breast cancer, conventionally trained doctors use tamoxifen or other anti-hormone drugs.

Unfortunately, those drugs only work for about 30 per cent of women whose tumours have oestrogen receptors and for about 70 per cent of women whose tumours have receptors for both oestrogen and progesterone. On top of that, women who take tamoxifen are two to three times more likely to develop endometrial cancer than women who are not on the drug *(Sadovsky, Richard, MD. Endometrial cancer in women receiving tamoxifen. American Family Physician. 1 January 2000)*.

Other serious side effects include the early onset of menopause, blood clots, strokes, uterine cancer and cataracts *(National Cancer Institute. Tamoxifen: Questions and Answers. http://www.cancer.gov;*

Chemicals known to the state to cause cancer or reproductive toxicity. State of California Environmental Protection Agency. 21 March 2008).

Although the combination of Aromasin and Avemar came out on top, taking Aromasin can cause harmful side effects including hair loss, constipation, hot flushes, vomiting, chest pain, depression, vision or speech changes, and nervous system disorders *(Aromasin side effects. Drugs.com. 4 June 2008).*

Although Avemar does not cause any adverse effects, American BioSciences does offer one caution. Because Avemar is a wheat product, there is a possibility of an allergic reaction, so people who are sensitive to gluten or wheat germ should not use Avemar.

- **New research shows pomegranate compounds kill breast cancer cells – but beware, many pomegranate supplements are a complete waste of money**

There are numerous health benefits linked to antioxidant-rich pomegranates. Their ability to fight heart disease and arthritis, and combat the effects of ageing has been well documented in recent years.

Now, the latest exciting research findings have revealed yet another benefit linked to this remarkable fruit… scientists have discovered that specific pomegranate compounds are able to stop the proliferation of breast cancer cells.

However, worrying new research has revealed that many pomegranate supplements currently lining the shelves of health food stores up and down the country are not the real deal. They contain little, if any, of the active ingredients responsible for many of the fruit's health benefits… including its ability to help fight cancer.

Don't worry, we've discovered a reputable pomegranate supplement that guarantees you're getting the real thing. But more on that later.

First, let's take a closer look at the latest research results on its breast cancer-fighting properties...

Preliminary findings are extremely promising...

Pomegranates are a rich source of natural chemicals called ellagitannins. When digested, these are broken down in the body into other chemicals, including ellagic acid, gallagic acid and urolithins A and B.

In the first of the two new studies, researchers at the University of California, Los Angeles, tested the ability of ellagitannin-derived compounds to block the conversion of sex hormones called androgens into oestrogen, which fuels the growth of some types of breast cancer *(Cancer Prev Res (Phila Pa) 2010 Jan; 3(1): 108-113)*. They also looked at how well the same pomegranate compounds directly inhibited the growth of oestrogen-responsive breast cancer cells in the laboratory.

They found that urolithin B had the strongest activity, both in blocking hormone conversion and in inhibiting cancer cell proliferation. The researchers concluded that "pomegranate ellagitannin-derived compounds have potential for the prevention of oestrogen-responsive breast cancers".

The second laboratory-based study investigated the effect of an omega-5 long-chain fatty acid in pomegranate seeds, called punicic acid, on the growth of both oestrogen-responsive and oestrogen-insensitive breast cancers *(Int J Oncol 2010 Feb; 36(2): 421-426)*.

This research, at the University of Minnesota, in the US, found that punicic acid inhibited the proliferation of both types of cancer by an amazing 96 per cent and 92 per cent respectively, compared with untreated controls. It also increased the rate of apoptosis, or 'cell suicide' by 91 per cent in oestrogen-responsive tumours, and by 86 per cent in the oestrogen-insensitive kind.

Beware of misleading claims on pomegranate products

As already mentioned, not all pomegranate supplements are the same, and it's difficult to know what you are getting from looking at the label on the bottle. Most of the supplements available are standardised to a minimum of 40 per cent ellagic acid. This may sound like a guarantee of effectiveness, but the shocking truth is that pomegranates naturally contain almost no ellagic acid.

Ellagic acid is actually produced in our bodies as a breakdown product of the ellagitannins present in pomegranates. Because ellagic acid was a compound that showed promise in early test-tube studies, it is still used as a quality standard for supplements and is meant to represent the amount that could, in theory, be produced once the supplement has been digested.

The trouble is that this means of standardising pomegranate supplements has led some unscrupulous manufacturers to add purified ellagic acid from cheaper sources to their products in order to claim '40 per cent ellagic acid content'. However, it is the synergistic action of the mix of ellagitannins present in the whole fruit that delivers pomegranate's anti-cancer and antioxidant benefits, rather than its actual or theoretical ellagic acid content *(Altern Med Rev 2008; 13(2): 128-144)*.

Such dirty dealing by supplement manufacturers is not uncommon, according to a 2009 study that analysed the contents of 27 pomegranate supplements available in America. Staggeringly, only five of these had the expected ellagitannin profile of whole pomegranate; 17 had ellagic acid as the main ingredient and little or no ellagitannin; while the remaining five contained neither ellagitannins nor ellagic acid! *(J. Agric. Food Chem 2009; 57: 7395–7400)*

When you choose a pomegranate supplement, it's important to pick one that is an extract of the whole fruit in its natural form and has not been bulked up with ellagic acid from other sources. Solgar Pomegranate Complex features a proprietary pomegranate extract from organically grown pomegranates, which is standardised for punicalagins rather than ellagic acid, and which contains exactly the same ellagitannins and other polyphenols, in the same proportions, as found in fresh pomegranates.

What to take for best results

The recommended dose of Solgar Pomegranate Complex is three vegetable capsules daily, preferably at mealtimes.

Chapter Five: Skin Cancer

The lowdown on skin cancer... could your sunscreen be doing you more harm than good?

During the summer months we are continually bombarded by the same message – 'don't go out without sunscreen, cover yourself up, or you risk getting skin cancer'. But, with sunscreen products providing multi-billion pound sales for the pharmaceutical and cosmetics industries, it's often hard to know where sound science ends and the marketing hype begins.

Skin cancer is one of the most common cancers in the UK, with the number of cases doubling in the past 20 years. Around 100,000 cases of skin cancer are diagnosed in the UK each year, 7,000 of which are the most dangerous kind, malignant melanoma (see the box below for details of the three main types of skin cancer).

Although we are constantly told that avoiding the sun's rays and using sunscreen will reduce our risk of this dreaded disease, the truth is not that simple and indeed the very opposite may in fact be true.

The 3 main types of skin cancer and how to spot them

1. Basal cell carcinoma – this is the most common form of skin cancer, which occurs most frequently in men who spend a lot of time outdoors. It is identifiable by lumps or patches that usually appear on the head or neck. You should seek your doctor's advice immediately if you spot any of these signs, caught early it does not pose too much of a risk as it rarely spreads to other parts of the body.

2. Squamous cell carcinoma – usually affects fair-skinned people with red or blonde hair, who burn easily and find it hard to get a tan.

It can cause an itchy, red, scaly patch of skin or a lump or sore. Again, early diagnosis is vital, especially in this case, as squamous cell carcinoma can spread to other parts of the body if left untreated.

3. Malignant melanoma – the rarest but also the most dangerous type of skin cancer. Worrying new figures from Cancer Research UK show a steep increase in deaths from malignant melanoma, especially in elderly men. In the late 1970s fewer than 400 (1.5 per 100,000) men died from melanoma but that figure has now risen to over 1,100 (3.1 per 100,000). It often grows from an existing mole, so make sure you check yours regularly and see your doctor straight away if you notice any changes such as bleeding, discolouration, enlargement or itchiness. It spreads rapidly to other organs and can be fatal if not treated early. Surprisingly, it often occurs on parts of the body not exposed to the sun and is most common in people who work indoors.

The sun produces your body's own defence against skin cancer – vitamin D

According to researchers at the Leiden University Medical Center in the Netherlands, lifetime sun exposure may be associated with an increased risk of the non-melanoma kinds of skin cancer, such as basal cell carcinoma and squamous cell carcinoma (*J Invest Dermatol 2003; 120: 1087-1093*). However, this is at odds with earlier research, which found no such link (*Cancer Causes and Controls 1994; 5: 367-392*).

In addition, the Leiden University study found that while lifetime sun exposure is linked to an increased risk of non-melanoma kinds of skin cancer it is also linked to a reduced risk of malignant melanoma. Dr Marianne Berwick at the University of New Mexico, has shown that spending frequent short periods of time in the sun is linked to a reduced risk of death from this form of the disease (*J Nat Cancer Inst 2005; 97: 195-199*).

This apparent protective effect of sun exposure may be because sunshine on our skin produces vitamin D. It has long been known that this vitamin suppresses the growth of malignant melanoma cells in the laboratory *(Endocrinology 1981; 108: 1083-1086)*. In addition, malignant melanoma patients are often found to be deficient in the active form of vitamin D (1,25-dihydroxyvitamin D3) that is generated by sun exposure *(Clin Cancer Res 2000; 2: 498-504)*.

New research questions the safety of many common ingredients found in sunscreens

Even if sun exposure does increase some skin cancer risks, can sunscreen creams really protect us? Some studies have found a link between the regular use of sunscreens and a lower incidence of cell changes, called actinic keratoses, which may precede squamous cell carcinoma *(JAMA 1994; 271(21): 1662-1663)*. However, there is no clear evidence that they protect us against basal cell carcinoma or malignant melanoma. In fact, sunscreens have been linked with an increased risk of these two forms of cancer *(Brit J Dermatol 2002; 146: 24)*.

This could be because sunscreen use encourages longer, more intense bouts of sunbathing, which appear to be more of a skin cancer risk than 'little and often' sun exposure *(BMJ 1994; 308: 75-76)*.

Or it may be because sunscreens block the UVB ultraviolet rays that produce vitamin D and so remove a natural anti-cancer mechanism. There is also evidence that it is the UVA rays, which many sunscreens hardly block at all, that can be a major factor in the development of malignant melanoma *(New England J Med 1999; 340: 1341-1348)*.

But most worrying of all is the possibility that the chemicals in sunscreens could themselves be a cause of skin cancer. For example, regular use of sunscreens that contain the chemical psoralen more than doubles the risk of skin cancer on average and increases it four and a half times for people who don't tan easily *(Int J Cancer 1995; 61: 749-755)*.

Another sunscreen chemical, called PBSA, was found to damage DNA in laboratory tests and the sunscreen chemical octyl methoxycinnamate (which is in more than 90 per cent of sunscreens) quickly kills animal cells exposed to light *(Chem Res Toxicol 1999; 12(1): 38-45; New Scientist 2000; 7 October: 13)*.

How to protect your skin during the summer months

- DON'T expose your skin to the sun for extended periods, with or without sunscreen – if you have to be outside for a long time, wear a hat and loose clothing.

- DON'T cover yourself with sunscreen – if you must use it to prevent burning, use it sparingly on areas most likely to burn. In addition, check the label for potentially harmful chemicals – like psoralen – which, as already mentioned, are actually linked to increasing the risk of certain types of skin cancer.

- DO aim to get frequent, moderate exposure to the sun (without sunscreen) – how much will depend on your skin type, time of year and geographical location – this will boost your vitamin D production.

- EAT more curry! This may sound like a strange bit of advice but US researchers from the University of Texas in Houston found that curcumin – the yellow pigment found in the curry spice turmeric – suppresses the growth of malignant melanoma cells in the laboratory *(Cancer 2005; 104(4): 879-890)*. You can also take curcumin in supplement form – take 900mg a day as a preventive measure.

- TAKING certain nutritional supplements may act as preventatives in the development of skin cancer. According to recent research, antioxidants – particularly beta-carotene, vitamin E and selenium – may prevent and counteract the sun-induced skin damage that can lead to skin cancer *(Photoderm, Photoimmunol, Photomed*

2004; 20: 297-304). Take 25,000 IU of beta-carotene, 400 IU of vitamin E and 200mcg of selenium daily.

Lutein is another antioxidant that could prevent the development of skin cancer. A study in which mice had the sensitive skin on their ears exposed to ultraviolet light found that those fed a diet supplemented with lutein experienced less cell damage *(J Invest Dermatol 2004; 122: 510-517)*. The recommended dosage is 4mg of lutein a day.

• VitaCell can protect your skin from sun-related damage – helping to lower your risk of skin cancer and wrinkles

When your skin is exposed to sunlight – and this can occur when skiing or working outdoors, not just on a hot beach – your body uses dietary antioxidants as well as natural pigmentation as part of its own protective mechanisms. If your dietary intake of antioxidants is compromised due to a busy lifestyle and a lack of fruit and vegetables, then it's a good idea to consider taking a supplement that tops up your levels of skin-friendly antioxidants, especially before going on holiday.

This is where a new formula called VitaCell can help – it contains a combination of nutrients and plant extracts that have been proven to maintain skin health, especially during periods of excessive sun exposure.

The product is based on lycopene and beta-carotene – antioxidants known as carotenoids which play a role in reducing skin sensitivity to UV radiation. It also contains vitamins C and E, selenium and green tea which are all potent antioxidants; zinc, which supports skin growth and repair; and beta-1,3 glucan, limonene and curcumin noted for their immune-supportive properties.

Lycopene and beta-carotene can reduce your risk of sunburn

Tomatoes, guava, rosehip, watermelon and pink grapefruit all get their red hue from lycopene. In the body, this antioxidant is deposited in your liver, lungs, prostate gland, colon and skin, and its concentration in tissues tends to be higher than all other carotenoids.

More and more research is emerging regarding lycopene's ability to protect the skin from sun damage. In one study, to establish whether eating 55g of tomato paste daily (providing 16mg of lycopene) for 12 weeks could help protect the skin from UV damage and UV-induced reddening, results showed that there was a 30 per cent increase in skin protection compared to those who did not consume the tomato paste *(Experimental Biology and Medicine 2002; 227: 845-851).*

Beta-carotene, which is a precursor to vitamin A, appears to decrease sensitivity to the sun, which could be of particular benefit to people with skin conditions caused by sunlight exposure, such as erythropoietic protoporphyria (an enzyme deficiency disorder).

One controlled study showed that taking carotenoids in supplement form (mainly beta-carotene) in daily amounts of 30mg, 60mg, and 90mg provided progressively more protection against ultraviolet rays *(Proc Soc Exp Biol Med 2000; 223: 170–4).* According to the findings of US researchers from the Mayo Clinic, lycopene in combination with other carotenoids, such as beta-carotene, may help reduce sunburn *(www.mayoclinic.org).*

Vitamin C, E and selenium help minimise the damage caused by harmful UV rays

Vitamin C is one of the best known antioxidants and is vital for collagen synthesis in your skin and tissue repair. Studies have revealed that levels of vitamin C in tissues exposed to UV radiation are reduced.

According to several double-blind studies, vitamin C (2,000-3,000mg daily) in combination with the antioxidant vitamin E (1,000 to 2,000 IU per day) have demonstrated a significant protective effect against UV rays *(Arch Dermatol 1994; 130: 1257–61; Free Radic Biol Med 1998; 25: 1006–12; J Am Acad Dermatol 1998; 38:45–8).*

Another study using combined antioxidants found that taking vitamin E and selenium (along with beta-carotene and lycopene) daily for seven weeks provided protection against ultraviolet light *(Photodermatol Photoimmunol Photomed 2003; 19: 182–9).*

Green tea and zinc – a powerful defence against sun-related skin damage

Green tea is rich in compounds known as polyphenols that have antioxidant and anti-inflammatory properties. In relation to UV exposure, ingestion of standardised green tea extract reduced or inhibited oedema, DNA damage, the growth rate of existing skin tumours and dermal penetration of UV radiation *(J Invest Dermatol 1999 Dec; 113(6): 1070-5; Arch Dermatol Res 2005 Apr; 296(10): 473-81; J Photochem Photobiol B. 2001 Dec 31; 65(2-3): 109-14).*

Zinc has been added to the VitaCell formulation because it aids tissue renewal and is required for the general maintenance of your skin.

UV radiation produces DNA strand breaks in exposed cells resulting in cell death (apoptosis). In one study, zinc supplementation significantly decreased apoptosis and the researchers concluded that the mineral was of significant interest for skin protection against UV radiation *(Biol Trace Elem Res 1999 Sep; 69(3): 177-90).* Interestingly, decreased levels of zinc have been noted in patients suffering from light sensitive skin conditions *(Dermatologica 1984; 169(2): 66-9).*

Beta-1,3 glucan, limonene and curcumin help boost immunity

Beta-1,3 glucan is a polysaccharide derived from the cell walls of oat kernels. It has a wide range of therapeutic applications including modulating the immune system and preventing cancer. It has been found to protect the body against various forms of radiation, which it does by scavenging cellular breakdown caused by these emissions. Some forms of radiation it protects against are from airline travel, X-rays, mammograms and UV rays from the sun.

Beta-1,3 glucan also helps regenerate and repair tissues, thereby accelerating the recovery of damaged skin cells.

Like beta-1,3 glucan, limonene has been incorporated into VitaCell as it has significant potential to modulate the immune response, which can be compromised by excess sun exposure.

As mentioned on page 45, the major active extract in the spice turmeric, curcumin is known for its antioxidant, anti-tumour and anti-inflammatory properties. In one study, curcumin effectively inhibited the uncontrolled spread of skin cancer cells.

What to take for best results

The recommended dosage for VitaCell is one capsule taken daily with food. If taking as a skin-protective supplement before going on holiday, it's best to take one capsule daily for six weeks before going, and then to continue supplementing throughout the holiday period.

Please be aware that VitaCell is not a replacement for other forms of sun protection such as sunscreen and a hat.

Contraindications: VitaCell is not suitable for individuals taking anti-blood clotting medication such as warfarin, heparin, coumarin or aspirin. This product should also be avoided during pregnancy and breastfeeding.

- ## Natural protection against sun damage – from the inside out!

Another cutting-edge natural product in the sun-protection arena, is SPF Skin Pro-Factors. This supplement has been specially formulated to aid in the maintenance of healthy skin, especially during the summer months. As already reported, overexposure to ultraviolet (UV) radiation from the sun increases the risk of skin cancer, ageing and eye cataracts.

SPF Skin Pro-Factors works on defending the skin from the inside by boosting UV protection, neutralising harmful free radicals created by UV exposure, and helping to prevent sunburn. The product contains four active ingredients: GliSODin®, astaxanthin, beta-carotene and grape seed extract.

The 'enzyme of life' reduces skin damage from ultraviolet rays

GliSODin® is a patented form of the enzyme SOD (superoxide dismutase), also known as 'the enzyme of life'. Naturally present both inside and outside cell membranes, SOD is one of the body's front line antioxidant enzyme defences and plays a critical role in reducing the rate of cell destruction caused by harmful free radicals. SOD levels normally decrease with age, while the body's susceptibility to free radical production increases, making the cells more vulnerable to degeneration.

Although SOD supplements have been used in an attempt to boost SOD levels in the body, research has found that oral SOD preparations are unlikely to have this effect. This is because the SOD protein molecule is easily deactivated by the powerful acids and enzymes in the digestive tract. However, with the creation of SOD in the form of GliSODin®, this obstacle appears to have been overcome.

GliSODin® is derived from French cantaloupe melon, which is a rich and valuable source of this potent antioxidant. To provide an effective means of transport and delivery through the gastrointestinal tract, this form of SOD is combined with a wheat gliadin polymer, which protects the SOD from being broken down and destroyed. Research reveals that supplementation with GliSODin® results in a significant increase in circulating antioxidant levels and significantly lower levels of free radical induced DNA damage.

According to studies, daily GliSODin® supplementation can significantly reduce UV damage, particularly in fair-skinned individuals *(Mac-Mary M, Sainthillier J, Creidi P, Series JP, Vix F, Humbert P. Evaluation of the Effect of Glisodin on the Intensity of Actinic Erythema. Annual Congress for Dermatological Research in Brest, France, May 2005)*. Researchers at the Besançon University Hospital in France carried out a randomised, double-blind, placebo-controlled study of the effects of GliSODin® intake in relation to UV skin protection.

The investigators used UV light to induce sunburn on the forearms of 50 subjects once a week for four weeks. Two to three days before the first irradiation, the participants took a daily supplement containing either GliSODin® or a placebo, which they continued to take throughout the study period. The researchers then used special instruments to measure skin colour and inflammatory changes in the skin.

Those in the GliSODin®-supplemented group experienced significant protection against UV exposure and also had less skin inflammation compared to the placebo group. "This study confirms the efficacy of GliSODin® in the prevention of the consequences of oxidative stress resulting from exposure to the sun," the researchers said.

Internal sunscreen that promotes more youthful skin

Astaxanthin is a carotenoid compound present in certain types of algae, where it protects these organisms from being destroyed by harsh sunlight.

The pigments, which stop algae from being damaged by the sun, also seem to protect human skin in the same way. Scientists believe that when astaxanthin is used as a supplement, it creates a natural protective barrier in the skin against UV rays – effectively working as an 'internal sunscreen'.

Research to date reveals that naturally-sourced algal astaxanthin helps prevent the DNA alterations that can be caused by ultraviolet 'A' radiation, and also reduces the pain and inflammation that occurs with sunburn *(J Dermatol Sci 2002 Oct; 30(1): 73-84)*.

With its ability to protect the skin from the sun, it's no surprise that astaxanthin functions as a powerful antioxidant. Laboratory comparisons show that it is 10 times more potent than beta-carotene in preventing free radical damage, and up to 550 times more effective as an antioxidant than vitamin E *(Pure Appl Chem 1991; 63: 141-146; Biochem Soc Trans 1990; 18: 1054 1056; Am J Clin Nutr 1991; 53: 194S-200S; Fisheries Science 1996; 62(1): 134-137)*.

Although the antioxidant beta-carotene is not as potent as astaxanthin, research has confirmed that this carotenoid compound can offer protection against sunburn, and the longer the supplementation period, the greater the protection. Another great benefit of beta-carotene is that it's converted by the body into vitamin A, which is essential for healthy skin and can actually help reduce age spots.

Wolfgang Kopcke and colleagues from Münster University Hospital, Germany, conducted a meta-analysis of seven studies which looked at the effect of supplementation with beta-carotene on sunburn in humans *(Photochem Photobiol 2008 Mar-Apr; 84(2): 284-288)*. They concluded that beta-carotene's sun protection factor (SPF) is about four and its probable mechanism of action is via its antioxidant activity.

When exposed to ultraviolet 'B' radiation, free radicals are produced in the skin that can lead to cell damage. Beta-carotene's antioxidant properties neutralise these reactive molecules, thereby offering skin protection.

Grape seed extract has been added to SPF Skin Pro-Factors as it protects against free radical damage, believed to be a major cause of the ageing process. It also works by reinforcing the collagen matrix of connective tissue and inhibiting collagen damage caused by inflammation and infection. Research suggests that grape seed extract promotes youthful skin, helps to protect the body from sun damage, and improves blood circulation by strengthening capillaries, arteries and veins *(J Med Food 2003 Winter; 6(4): 291-299)*.

Besides its role in protecting the skin from sun damage, SPF Skin Pro-Factors may be useful for easing acne, inflammatory skin conditions and autoimmune diseases affecting skin health such as lupus (SLE). It can also be taken as a general antioxidant supplement and to improve skin health.

What to take for best results

The recommended dosage for SPF Skin Pro-Factors is one to three capsules daily. If using for skin protection while on holiday, you should ideally take the product at least two weeks before travelling to build up tissue levels, and then daily during the period of sun exposure.

Due to the presence of the wheat protein gliadin, SPF Skin Pro-Factors is not recommended for use by people with coeliac disease or anyone who is wheat or gluten intolerant/allergic. It should also be avoided during pregnancy and lactation.

Chapter Six: Colon Cancer

Colon cancer, also known as rectal, colorectal or bowel cancer, affects the lower part of the digestive system – the large bowel and the rectum. It affects men and women equally, and is the third most common type of cancer in men and the second most common in women.

Each year, more than 35,000 people are diagnosed with colon cancer and about 16,000 die as a result of the disease. It is not easy to treat, mainly because it's often detected only once well-established – and possibly spread beyond the bowel itself.

However, estimates suggest that nine out of 10 colon cancers detected early can be successfully treated. That's why it's important to recognise the symptoms, which can easily be mistaken for less life-threatening complaints such as piles or irritable bowel syndrome. Doctors advise that if the following symptoms persist for longer than a couple of weeks, you should seek medical attention straight away:

- Blood flecks in your stools, particularly if the blood is dark or plum-coloured. This is the most commonly noticed symptom and should never be ignored.
- A change in your regular bowel habits, such as constipation or diarrhoea, that's severe or lasts for two weeks or more.
- A feeling that you need to empty your bowels even when you have just been to the toilet.
- Abdominal pain or discomfort that lasts for two weeks or more.
- Unexplained weight loss.
- Some people feel tired, dizzy or breathless because they've become anaemic from microscopic bleeding from the bowel.

Colon cancer screening: new non-invasive method investigated

To diagnose colon cancer, your doctor may perform a rectal examination to check for any abnormal changes. This involves putting a gloved finger in your rectum to feel for any lumps or swellings.

In 2006 the government introduced the NHS bowel cancer screening programme. It offers routine screening every two years to all men and women aged 60 to 69 (50 to 74 in Scotland).

To investigate bowel cancer symptoms, doctors and hospital specialists often ask patients to undergo sigmoidoscopy or colonoscopy. Both involve gently pushing a long thin tube containing a tiny video camera through your back passage and into the rectum and colon to take a close look at the inside of your bowel. If polyps or abnormal areas of the lining of the bowel are seen, biopsies may be taken and sent to the laboratory for analysis. This can be uncomfortable, but is very seldom a painful experience.

For more than three decades, optical colonoscopy (OC) has been the primary method of colon cancer screening. But an alternative method called computed tomographic colonography (CTC) has been developed over the past few years. This method is also known as 'virtual colonoscopy' because it's minimally invasive, requiring a catheter to be inserted into the rectum to fill the colon with air, followed by a non-invasive optical scan.

Researchers at the University of Wisconsin Medical School, in the US, set out to discover whether CTC is as effective as OC *(New England Journal of Medicine, Vol. 357, No. 14, 10/4/07):*

- The researchers compared screening results from 3,163 patients who underwent traditional colonoscopy to the results from 3,120 patients who were examined with the CTC technique.

- In the CTC screening, 123 advanced tumours were found, compared to 121 in the OC group.
- Total polyps removed in the CTC group: 561.
- Total polyps removed in the OC group: 2,434.
- Seven perforations of the colon occurred in the OC group compared to none in the CTC group.

The researchers concluded: "These findings support the use of CTC as a primary screening test before therapeutic OC."

The risk of a perforated colon is a clear drawback for traditional colonoscopy, but let's take another look at two of those bullet points regarding the total polyps removed. Those numbers are so lopsided because all polyps are routinely removed on the spot during OC, but when polyps were detected in the CTC group, patients were given the option of leaving very small polyps in place or undergoing an additional OC procedure to remove the polyps.

Tiny polyps may never become a problem, but with OC there's no question – the polyps are removed. The importance of managing the development of colon polyps can't be overstated. When pre-cancerous polyps are removed, the risk of developing colorectal cancer is sharply reduced. And this is a clear advantage of traditional colonoscopy. In the University of Wisconsin study, about eight per cent of the patients underwent follow-up OC after undergoing CTC.

One benefit of the CTC procedure is that, according to a HealthDay report about a 2005 study of 500 patients who underwent CTC, in more than half the cases doctors discovered other health issues that were unrelated to the colon – problems such as lesions, masses in solid organs, and large aneurysms. If you're due for a colon screening, talk to your doctor about the pros and cons of the CTC and OC techniques.

A barium enema may also be carried out. This involves injecting a dye into the lower bowel via an enema, which shows up on X-rays to help doctors' spot signs of cancers. If the diagnosis is cancer, the tumour will then be 'staged'. Doctors may order more complex tests such as scans (CT or MRI), to check to see if the cancer has spread to involve other organs such as the liver. It helps doctors to work out what treatment is most appropriate.

What happens if you're diagnosed with colon cancer?

The main option for treating colon cancer is surgery, and if the disease can be caught before it breaks through the bowel wall, the patient's chances are much higher. Usually, the piece of bowel that contains the cancer is removed and the two open ends are joined back together. This operation is called a bowel 'resection' by doctors.

If the two sections can't be joined back together, often because the tumour is too low, the bowel can be brought out through the abdominal wall. This is called a stoma, which is connected to a colostomy bag. Although this procedure is more likely after removal of a tumour in the rectum, it's not always necessary and may only be temporary.

Chemotherapy and radiotherapy are increasingly being used to treat colon cancer in addition to surgery, especially in cases where tumours are advanced. For example, a combination of radiotherapy and chemotherapy may be given before surgery for rectal cancer. This is known as neoadjuvant therapy, and it may reduce the risk of recurrence and improve survival rates.

How well patients do after treatment depends on the stage that the cancer has reached. Survival rates have improved in the past 30 years but overall survival is still only about 50 per cent at five years. However, when colon cancer is caught early – before it has spread to other organs such as the liver or the lungs – the chances of recovery are high, more than 80 per cent.

Colon cancer: Are you at risk?

Your chances of developing colon cancer increase if:

- A close relative (sibling or parent) has had colon polyps or has been diagnosed with colorectal cancer.
- You're over the age of 65. The disease is rare in people under 40 and almost 85 per cent of cases are diagnosed in over 65 year olds.
- You smoke.
- You drink alcohol.
- You exercise infrequently or not at all.
- Your diet is high in processed foods and low in fibre, fruit and veg.
- You have had previous problems with chronic inflammatory bowel disease, such as long standing ulcerative colitis or Crohn's disease.

How elevated levels of C-reactive protein could spell colon cancer

C-reactive protein is produced by your liver in response to inflammation. Over the years, researchers have found high levels of CRP to be associated with various chronic health problems, including stroke, heart disease and diabetes.

A team headed by researchers at the Johns Hopkins Bloomberg School of Public Health in the US, reported on a population-based study designed to see if there's a link between elevated CRP levels and colorectal cancer.

Researchers used data collected from a study called CLUE II (named for a campaign called 'Give Us a Clue to Cancer and Heart Disease'), conducted in Maryland. The records of nearly 23,000 adults included blood tests and health questionnaires. Additional data was gathered on the subjects for more than 10 years.

The Hopkins team identified 172 cases of colorectal cancer, and compared the data for these cases against 342 control subjects who were cancer-free, but matched the cancer subjects by age, sex and race.

The results showed that CRP levels were about the same among those with rectal cancer and subjects in the control group. But researchers determined that CRP levels were significantly higher among those with colon cancer. Overall, the highest levels of CRP indicated double the risk of developing colorectal cancer and two and a half times the risk of colon cancer, compared with subjects with the lowest CRP levels.

Because CRP levels can be measured with a simple blood test, this inflammation marker is quickly becoming one of the most critical tools in assessing risk of chronic health problems. So the next time you have a physical examination, ask your doctor to check your CRP. If it's elevated, and if you also have a family history of colorectal cancer, your doctor will probably suggest that you have a colonoscopy examination – especially if you're over the age of 50.

Obviously, some risk factors, such as age and having a family history of the disease, can't be altered. But, one risk factor you can alter is your diet... the importance of nutrition when it comes to lowering the risk of colon cancer can't be emphasised enough, as the following research findings show...

• Eating plenty of fibre can help ward off colon cancer

Exciting new research findings have just become available, following the largest study ever to be undertaken regarding the link between diet and colon cancer. Researchers from the European Prospective Investigation into Cancer (EPIC) found that individuals who consume the highest amount of fibre in their diets have almost half the risk of colon cancer than those who consume only low amounts.

These findings knock on the head the results of a similar, smaller-scale US trial, also carried out recently, which concluded that fibre "may not prevent bowel cancer" – news that the media was quick to leap on.

However, it was noted by the American Institute for Cancer Research that the US study, which found no association between fibre intake and colon cancer incidence in women, involved a population with low fibre intake. Women who consumed the highest amounts of fibre in this study had intakes equivalent to those in the EPIC study's low fibre group.

The EPIC study followed a massive 519,978 European participants, aged between 24 and 75, from 10 countries, for four and a half years. During this period 1,065 cases of colon cancer were diagnosed. The researchers discovered that those whose dietary fibre consumption was in the top 20 per cent, at 35g per day, experienced a 40 per cent lower risk of developing colon cancer than individuals who consumed an average of 15g per day.

Another recent study showed similar results. Researchers involved in The Prostate, Lung, Colorectal and Ovarian Cancer Screening Trial, found that patients who had the highest dietary fibre intakes, had a 27 per cent lower risk of developing polyps than those patients who ate very little fibre. Polyps are benign mushroom-shaped growths that can grow over time and become cancerous – colon polyps are frequently precursors of colon cancer.

Reporting on these two large-scale trials in *The Lancet*, authors Lynnette Ferguson and Philip Harris of the University of Auckland, New Zealand, write: "Whatever the reasons for the results reported by the two studies, eating a diet rich in plant foods, in the form of fruit, vegetables, and whole-grain cereals, probably remains the best option for reducing the risk of colon cancer, and for more general health protection."

In addition, beans, nuts and seeds are also rich sources of fibre – so make sure you include plenty in your diet.

• Men – lower your risk of colorectal cancer by eating more calcium and dairy

Researchers from the Karolinska Institute in Stockholm, Sweden found that men whose diets were high in calcium and dairy had a lower risk of developing colorectal cancer *(Am J Clin Nutr 2006; 83(3): 667-73).*

In 1997, the scientists enrolled 45,306 men who had no history of cancer and were between the ages of 45 to 79. They kept track of these volunteers for an average of 6.7 years. The men completed food frequency questionnaires at the beginning of the study and these were analysed by the researchers for calcium and dairy intake.

During the study 276 volunteers were diagnosed with colon cancer and 173 with rectal cancer. The researchers found that the men whose calcium intake was in the top one-fourth of all the volunteers had a 32 per cent lower risk of developing colorectal cancer. For dairy foods, consuming seven or more servings a day reduced the risk to 54 per cent when compared to the men who ate less than two servings a day.

This study suggests that dairy has the greatest protective effect on the colon. Commenting on the findings, the researchers said: "Future studies should examine the relation of other components of dairy foods, such as conjugated linoleic acid, sphingolipids, and milk proteins, with the risk of colorectal cancer."

So if you want to lower your risk of developing colorectal cancer, it may be worth making sure you get enough calcium, specifically from yoghurt and cheese. If you are looking to incorporate some non-dairy food sources of calcium, you can try some of these foods: green, leafy vegetables – including broccoli, collard greens, kale, mustard greens, turnip greens and pak choi or Chinese cabbage – canned salmon and sardines, shellfish, almonds, Brazil nuts and dried beans.

• Calcium may help prevent and treat polyps

Calcium intake has also been shown to help reduce the risk of developing colon polyps. Researchers from the Dartmouth-Hitchcock Medical Center in New Hampshire, US, published an analysis of data collected from 930 patients enrolled in the Calcium Polyp Prevention Study.

All of the study subjects had been diagnosed with colorectal polyps. Divided into two groups, participants received either a 1,200mg daily supplement of calcium carbonate, or a placebo. Two colonoscopies were conducted approximately one year and four years after each subject's initial examinations.

The researchers found that while calcium supplements may provide some protection against the development of polyps, the supplements proved most effective against advanced polyps. Subjects who received calcium supplements had generally fewer polyps compared to the placebo group. Dr John A Baron, lead researcher of the study, claimed calcium may help lower the risk of advanced polyps by as much as 45 per cent.

As US physician, and *HSI* Panellist, Dr Spreen notes: "Calcium is not found in nature (in edible form) without magnesium, and they therefore should always be given together."

Wholegrains, leafy green vegetables, beans, meat, bananas, apricots and nuts are all good sources of magnesium. Increasing your magnesium intake is a wise move, not only to ensure optimal calcium intake but also because it has been found to have its own anti-colon cancer benefits...

- **Animal studies indicate that dietary magnesium may protect against colon cancer**

Scientists at the Karolinska Institute in Stockholm, Sweden, gathered dietary and medical records on more than 61,000 women, aged 40 to 75 years, who were cancer-free at the outset of the study. Over a follow-up period of nearly 15 years, about 800 cases of colorectal cancer were diagnosed.

Analysis of the data showed that women with the highest dietary intake of magnesium reduced their risk of colorectal cancer by 40 per cent, compared to women who had the lowest magnesium intake. This association held true when data was broken down to reflect cases of colon cancer or rectal cancer.

Dietary magnesium is easy to come by. As mentioned earlier, the mineral is naturally present in green leafy vegetables, avocados, nuts and seeds, and whole grains, but usually in small amounts, so you need to eat a wide variety of these foods regularly to get all the magnesium you need.

Research indicates that many adults are not getting enough magnesium in their diets. This is largely due to the stresses on the body that deplete stores of magnesium. Starch, for instance, depletes magnesium, as does stress. You may also be at increased risk for magnesium deficiency if you regularly consume alcohol or diuretics because both can increase urinary excretion of the mineral. Prescription medications, like the antibiotics Gentamicin, Amphotericin, and Cyclosporin, can increase magnesium excretion as well.

If you're concerned that you might have a magnesium deficiency, ask your doctor to test your blood for magnesium levels. A normal range is anywhere between .66 and 1.23 mmol/L (millimoles per litre). Then you can be reassured that your magnesium intake is getting absorbed to deliver all the benefits from this essential nutrient.

Dr Allan Spreen recommends 500mg of magnesium a day, since absorption of most forms isn't that great anyway. His limit for oral magnesium is that which causes any loosening of the stools (and there's always a distinct dose that will do it... in fact, it works like a charm for constipated people by taking a known dose at bedtime, plus it helps them sleep).

Dr Spreen says he is careful to warn people not to go over that limit for the simple reason that food is moved through the GI tract too quickly with too much magnesium, and that cuts down on absorption of nutrients (both from foods and supplements). However, that amount is usually between 400 and 1,500mg/day.

- **These 5 key nutrients may prevent colorectal polyps from developing**

Researchers at a digestive cancer centre in Dijon, France, reported on a study in which colorectal polyp risk was compared to intake of dietary vitamins and beta-carotene (a plant chemical that the body converts into vitamin A).

Nutrient intakes were assessed in two groups: more than 360 subjects with polyps, and about 425 polyp-free subjects. The Dijon team found five nutrients that were associated with a lower risk of colorectal polyps: folate, beta-carotene, and vitamins B6, C and D.

But beta-carotene received a special note. Scientists are not yet sure why beta-carotene intake produces adverse effects among smokers. Previous research has shown that smokers are at higher risk of developing lung cancer when they have a large intake of beta-carotene and a low intake of other antioxidants.

In the Dijon study, data indicated that beta-carotene intake might increase colorectal polyp risk among smokers, while lowering risk

158

among non-smokers. The researchers suggest that smokers avoid high doses of beta-carotene.

---

4 simple ways to lower your risk of colon cancer

1. Up your intake of vitamin D. Following on from the Dijon study, another study has revealed that vitamin D may play an important role in the fight against colon cancer. The study involved more than 3,000 subjects, aged 50 to 75 years, who were screened for colon cancer. Using dietary questionnaires, researchers found a clear association between vitamin D intake of more than 645 IU per day and a reduced risk of colon cancer. Those who had the greatest protection also used multivitamins, exercised regularly, and had diets with a high fibre content. Moderate sun exposure, wild salmon and cod liver oil supplements are excellent sources of vitamin D. The Dijon research findings also back up point number 2…

2. Study after study attests to vitamin B6's colon cancer-fighting properties. A *JAMA* meta-analysis of 13 studies from Sweden's Karolinska Institute has revealed that high vitamin B6 intake and raised blood levels of PLP, the active form of B6, are linked to lower colorectal cancer risk — and the higher the PLP levels, the stronger the link (*"Vitamin B6 and Risk of Colorectal Cancer" Journal of the American Medical Association, Vol. 303, No. 11, 3/17/10, jama.ama-assn.org*).

For example:

- A Harvard Medical School study, in the US, showed that subjects with the highest B6 levels had a much lower risk of colorectal cancer compared to subjects with the lowest levels.

- Tufts University research found that even a modest deficiency of

---

key components in the B complex (including B6) increased colorectal cancer risk.

- In a large study conducted at the University of Edinburgh, high levels of B6 intake reduced colorectal cancer risk by more than 20 per cent.

- Another Harvard trial found colorectal cancer risk significantly reduced among subjects who had the highest dietary intake of folate and B6.

The two best sources of vitamin B6 are bananas and chicken breast meat. Fish, red meat, beans, and a wide variety of other plant foods also contain B6.

3. Don't underestimate the importance of a daily multivitamin. Multivitamin use was examined in a 2003 study conducted by the American Cancer Society. More than 145,000 subjects participated in the study that ran between 1992 and 1997. Researchers found that among subjects who began taking multivitamins just prior to the 1992 enrolment, there was no association with a reduced risk of colorectal cancer. But the participants who had reported regular multivitamin use (four or more times per week) in the early 1980s, fared much better: their group had a 30 per cent reduced risk of the cancer.

4. Getting your five a day is a must in the fight against colon cancer. A University of Minnesota study involving more than 1,700 subjects showed how a diet containing ample amounts of fruits and vegetables may be a significant factor in preventing pre-cancerous polyps from developing into cancer. Results also showed that women who drank the most fruit juice reduced their risk of developing polyps by half. The researchers speculate that the high folate intake from orange juice probably contributed to this resistance to polyp development. Why this 'juice effect' didn't hold true for men couldn't be answered by the researchers who carried out the study.

• Folic acid can help prevent cancerous colon polyps

Irish researchers have found that folic acid supplements can actively protect you from colon cancer. The good news is that the protective effect is most noticeable in people at highest risk of colon cancer – those who have been diagnosed with colon polyps (benign tumours that can become malignant over time).

A paper published in the journal *Gut* reported that folic acid acts to stop the proliferation of cells in the mucosa (lining) of the colon. If uncontrolled proliferation continues, it can lead to the development of adenomatous polyps that have the potential to become colon cancer.

In the Irish study, 20 patients with recurrent adenomatous polyps received 2mg of folic acid per day or a placebo for 12 weeks. Rectal biopsy samples were taken from the participants before supplementation, and at four, 12 and 18 weeks in order to examine cell proliferation. Blood samples were also taken.

The patients completed three-day dietary questionnaires at the study's onset and following supplementation, and the researchers calculated the amount and type of food consumed.

The researchers found that although mucosal cell proliferation between the groups was similar at the beginning of the study, the group receiving folic acid experienced a reduction in proliferation by the study's conclusion.

The most significant reduction took place at the upper aspect of the 'crypt'. Crypts are the indentations in the walls of the colon in which cells grow and replicate, with oldest cells existing at the top. Animal studies have shown that changes in mucosal crypt cells are related to colon cancer risk.

The researchers speculate that increasing folic acid may work by protecting DNA in individual mucosal cells from breakage and mutation. A deficiency of folate may also impair DNA repair in the mucosa of the colon and lead to chromosomal abnormalities at vulnerable sites.

You may want to take a combined folic acid and multivitamin pill on a daily basis. Alternatively, you should boost your diet with folic acid rich foods, such as leafy green vegetables (especially spinach), liver, yeast extract, wholegrains and freshly squeezed orange juice.

Chapter Seven: Bladder Cancer

B ladder cancer affects over 10,200 people every year in the UK, and is about three times more common in men than it is in women. It's rare in people under 40, but the rate rises with age.

Fortunately, bladder cancer is now considered one of the more survivable cancers, with more than half of both men and women alive five years after diagnosis.

Blood in your urine (haematuria) is the most common symptom of bladder cancer. This may come and go and is often painless.

Other symptoms include:

- a burning feeling when passing urine
- a need to pass urine frequently
- feeling the need to urinate but not being able to
- pain in your pelvis
- recurrent urinary tract infections
- blood clots in your urine (these may cause pain)

It's important that you visit your doctor if you experience any of these symptoms – but don't panic, they don't necessarily mean you have bladder cancer and often indicate the presence of non-malignant conditions such as urinary tract infections.

Causes of bladder cancer

At the moment, the causes of bladder cancer aren't fully understood. However, there are known risk factors, including:

- Smoking – you're three to four times more likely to develop bladder cancer if you smoke. More concerning is that passive smoking may also increase your risk.

- Exposure to certain industrial chemicals (e.g. in the rubber, paint, dye, printing and textile industries, gas and tar manufacturing, iron and aluminium processing).

- Increasing age. Most bladder cancers occur in people over the age of 50. It is rare in people younger than 40.

- Gender. As mentioned already, bladder cancer is about three times more common in men than women.

- Ethnic background. Bladder cancer is more common in white people than in black people.

- Previous radiotherapy or chemotherapy increases the risk.

- Schistosomiasis. This bladder infection, which is caused by a parasite in certain hot countries, increases the risk.

- Repeated bouts of other types of bladder infection may also slightly increase the risk.

How is bladder cancer diagnosed?

Urine microscopy – a sample of urine is sent to a laboratory to look for cancerous cells under a microscope. However, if no cancer cells are seen it does not rule out bladder cancer. Further tests are performed to confirm or rule out the diagnosis if symptoms suggest bladder cancer.

Cystoscopy – this test is commonly carried out to confirm a bladder tumour. A cystoscopy allows the urologist to look into your bladder with a special thin telescope called a cystoscope. The cystoscope is passed into the bladder via your urethra. A cystoscopy is normally carried out under local anaesthetic. However, if a procedure is performed via a cystoscope, such as removing a tumour, then a general anaesthetic is usually used.

During cystoscopy a urologist can:

- See any areas on the lining of the bladder which look abnormal.
- Take biopsies of suspicious areas. A biopsy is when a small sample of tissue is removed from a part of the body. The sample is then examined under the microscope to look for abnormal cells.
- Remove a superficial tumour with instruments which can be passed down a side channel of the cystoscope.

Special urine tests – urine tests have been developed which can detect bladder cancer, such as the BTA test, the NMP22 test and the Mcm5 test. These tests detect chemicals and proteins in urine that are made by bladder cancer cells. However, these tests are still not sensitive enough to diagnose all bladder cancers so are not routinely used.

Ultrasound scan – this safe and painless test uses sound waves to create images of organs and structures inside your body. It is sometimes used to diagnose bladder cancer.

CT scan – another test called CT urogram is a special type of CT scan that obtains pictures of your urinary tract. This is sometimes done to look for a bladder tumour.

If initial tests confirm that the cancer is a superficial tumour then no further tests may be necessary. Superficial bladder tumours have a low risk of spreading to other parts of the body.

However, if you have a muscle invasive tumour, then further tests, such as a CT or MRI scan, may be advised to assess if the cancer has spread. This assessment is called 'staging' of the cancer. The aim of staging is to find out:

- How much the tumour in the bladder has grown, and whether it has grown to the edge, or through the outer part of the bladder wall.

- Whether the cancer has spread to local lymph nodes.
- Whether the cancer has spread to other areas of the body (metastasised).

By finding out the stage of the cancer it helps doctors to advise on the best treatment options. It also gives a reasonable indication of outlook (prognosis).

Treating bladder cancer

Treatment very much depends on how far the cancer has spread.

A treatment called BCG, better known as a vaccine against TB, appears to work against bladder cancer cells, possibly because it helps stimulate the cells of the immune system to attack and kill cancer cells. However, its use is still predominantly experimental. About 50 per cent of superficial bladder cancer cases will return but most can be controlled quite easily with further surgery.

If it's confined to the lining of the bladder, then a simple procedure called transurethral resection (TUR) can be carried out. This is similar to cystoscopy, except the probe is used to burn away cancer cells with an electric current. This is normally carried out under general anaesthetic. The patient may have pain when passing urine for a short time afterwards, and some blood in the urine.

In about 20 per cent of cases the cancer will have invaded deeper into the tissues by the time of diagnosis, and in five per cent it will have spread further to another part of the body. These tumours are more difficult to treat. If the cancer has spread into the bladder muscle, then a bigger operation may be needed.

If the cancer is not particularly fast-spreading and aggressive, and is confined to only one part of the bladder wall, then a partial or 'segmental' cystectomy could be carried out. This involves removing part of the bladder, and allows the patient to urinate normally once recovered. However, if the cancer has spread more, 'radical' cystectomy is carried out, and the entire bladder is taken out, along with any nearby organs that bladder cancer cells may have spread to.

If the bladder has been removed, the patient no longer has anywhere to store the constant slow stream of urine coming from the kidneys. The surgeon creates an opening in the patient's side, which is called a stoma. This allows a bag to be attached to collect the urine.

A piece of the patient's own small intestine can be used as the tube carrying the urine to the stoma. Modern surgical techniques may allow a replacement bladder to be fashioned in some patients, giving back a degree of urinary control, and doctors are constantly improving these.

Your doctor may also recommend radiotherapy either as the first treatment, or to try to kill any cancer cells which remain after surgery. This is either targeted on the pelvic area, or given as a radioactive implant which is placed directly into the bladder.

Chemotherapy can also be directly targeted at the bladder in some cases, which helps prevent some of the unpleasant sideeffects, with drugs being pumped up a catheter via the urethra into the bladder. However, if the cancer is widely spread, then standard chemotherapy may be used to try to kill lingering cancer cells.

Immunotherapy – harnessing the immune system to fight bladder cancer, is also widely used in some cases of superficial cancer.

Only about 25 per cent of those with a local spread of the cancer will survive more than three years, and far fewer when the tumour has spread to other organs. Unfortunately, it's very difficult to predict who will be cured by treatment and when the cancer might recur.

As with all cancers, there are a number of research trials underway to look for more effective combinations of treatments, as well as trials of urine tests which might help to detect bladder cancer more easily.

New research findings offer hope in the fight against bladder cancer

New research published in *Cancer Causes and Control* has revealed that vitamin E, carotenoids (yellow, orange, and red pigments synthesized by plants), niacin, thiamine, and vitamin D may reduce the risk of bladder cancer in older people.

Researchers, led by Maree Brinkman from The Cancer Council Victoria in Australia, analysed dietary data from 322 people with bladder cancer and 239 healthy controls. A 121-item food frequency questionnaire was used to estimate dietary intakes.

Results of the study showed that, in general, people with the highest average intakes of vitamin E (at least 193.4mg per day) were 34 per cent less likely to develop bladder cancer. The highest average intakes of phosphorous (1,557mg) were associated with a 51 per cent reduction in bladder cancer risk.

When the researchers focused their analysis on smokers, they found that the highest intakes of vitamin E, carotenoids (18mg), and niacin (46.5mg), were associated with a 42, 38, and 34 per cent reduction in bladder cancer risk in heavy smokers.

In older individuals, the highest average intakes of carotenoids, vitamin D (641 IU), thiamine (3.35mg), niacin, and vitamin E were all associated with a reduced risk of bladder cancer.

The researchers made the following comment about their findings: "Bladder cancer is a disease that typically affects older people, and bioavailability of B-group vitamins may be compromised in this demographic by certain drugs (e.g. acid-lowering agents).

Additionally, vitamin E, like carotenoids acts as an antioxidant and, as suggested by our results, could be more beneficial under conditions of the greatest oxidative stress such as smoking and ageing."

Eat your way to a healthier bladder

Based on these findings, try to incorporate more of the following foods in your diet, which are rich sources of carotenoids, vitamin E, niacin, thiamine, and vitamin D.

Carotenoids: The most common carotenoids are alpha-carotene (carrots, winter squash, tomatoes, green beans, coriander and Swiss chard), beta-carotene (sweet potatoes, kale, spinach, turnip greens and fresh thyme), beta-cryptoxanthin (red bell peppers, papaya, coriander, oranges, corn and watermelon), lutein (kale, green peas, broccoli, papaya and egg), zeaxanthin (courgettes, corn, garden peas and Brussels sprouts), and lycopene (tomatoes, pink grapefruit, watermelon and guava).

Vitamin E: Foods rich in vitamin E are: wheat germ oil, almonds, sunflower seeds, sunflower oil, hazelnuts, spinach, broccoli, mango and tomato.

Niacin and Thiamine: Foods containing niacin (vitamin B3) and thiamine (vitamin B1) include: beef, pork, chicken, wheat flour, maize flour, eggs, milk, peas and roe.

Vitamin D: Whilst the best source of vitamin D is direct sunlight, those of us living in the northern hemisphere do sometimes fall short of this vital vitamin. The best concentrated food sources for vitamin D include salmon, sardines, shrimp, milk, cod and eggs.

How cruciferous vegetables can lower your risk of bladder cancer by up to 30%

Increasing your intake of cruciferous vegetables may slash your risk of bladder cancer by up to 30 per cent according to new research, which lays the benefits at the feet of their isothiocyanate content.

Epidemiological and animal studies have shown that diets high in cruciferous vegetables result in less instances of certain cancers especially lung, colon, breast and ovarian cancers… but no study up until now has reported on the risk reductions against bladder cancer.

The US study, carried out by researchers at the University of TexasMD Anderson Cancer Center, investigated the potential of dietary isothiocyanates to reduce the risk of bladder cancer. Diets were assessed using epidemiologic and food frequency questionnaires for 697 newly diagnosed bladder cancer cases and 708 healthy controls matched by age, gender and ethnicity.

The researchers found that the average daily intake of isothiocyanates was significantly lower in those with bladder cancer than for the healthy control subjects.

According to lead researcher Hua Zhao, the highest intake of isothiocyanates was associated with a 29 per cent reduction in bladder cancer risk compared to the lowest intake, with greater protection also observed in subjects over 64 years of age, men, and smokers.

The researchers suggest that the protective effects of the isothiocyanates against bladder cancer may be due to the increased exposure of the organ to the compounds – the majority of compounds produced by isothiocyanate metabolism are excreted through the urine.

The cancer-fighting properties of broccoli, a member of the cruciferous family of vegetables, are not new and previous studies have related these benefits to the high levels of active plant chemicals called glucosinolates. These are metabolised by the body into isothiocynates, and evidence suggests these are powerful anti-carcinogens. The main isothiocynate from broccoli is sulforaphane.

Chapter Eight: Cervical Cancer

Cervical dysplasia: Don't panic if your smear test result shows abnormalities... it doesn't necessarily spell cancer

I t's a moment every woman dreads – getting a smear test result that indicates the presence of 'abnormal cells'. Yet these fears often turn out to be groundless, as the test itself has been found to be largely unreliable. This is disturbing as it can result in women having dangerous surgery needlessly performed, when changes in cervical cells can usually be reversed back to normal simply by correcting vitamin deficiencies.

The cells lining the neck of the womb, or cervix, form layers – with young, round cells at the bottom, rising to the surface and flattening in shape as they mature. In cervical dysplasia (meaning 'abnormal growth'), some of these cells don't fit this pattern and grow at random anywhere within the layers.

Cells may also be described as 'atypical' when they appear irregular in shape, but are not abnormal enough to be called dysplasia. Cervical dysplasia is classified as 'mild' when only a few cells are abnormal; 'moderate' when about half the thickness of the layers of cells are affected; and 'severe' when the entire thickness contains abnormal cells.

The risk of cervical dysplasia developing into cancer is extremely small

Cervical dysplasia is not the same as cervical cancer and is confined to the very thin lining, or epithelium, that covers your cervix. On average, only one woman in every 625 who gets a negative smear test result develops cervical cancer, and 90 per cent of cases of cervical cancer can be treated successfully *(Lancet 342: 91-6, 1993)*.

Abnormal cells can be the result of inflammation due to a low-grade infection, which can occur in up to half the women tested *(Brit. Med. J. 306: 1173, 1993)*. Other studies have shown that about half of smears with 'mild' abnormalities revert to normal within two years and there is no steady progression from 'mild' to 'severe' dysplasia *(Brit. Med. J. 297: 18-21, 1988; Lancet, 339: 828, 1992)*.

In fact, very little is known about how cervical dysplasia or cervical cancer progress, which is why many doctors err on the side of caution and recommend early and aggressive treatment for dysplasia. But studies comparing early treatment with a 'wait and see' approach have shown that it makes no difference to the number of women who go on to develop cervical cancer – the ratio is still 1 in 625 *(Lancet 342: 91-6, 1993)*.

Having treatment to destroy abnormal cells or a 'cone' biopsy (in which a cone-shaped piece is cut from the cervix for examination), carries a risk of uncontrollable bleeding or permanent damage to your cervix. This can make sexual intercourse extremely painful, and also increases your chances of having a miscarriage if you become pregnant.

The accuracy of your smear test can depend on where you live!

An astonishing 50 per cent of smear test slides sent to laboratories are in effect useless because the sample has been taken incorrectly *(V Coleman, The Health Scandal: 172, 1988)*.

And at the laboratory, interpretation of the slides can differ widely. In some areas of England, nearly 20 per cent of smears are considered abnormal, compared with only 3 per cent in other areas *(Nat. Audit Office: Cervical and Breast Screening in England, 1992)*. So you may be told you have an 'abnormality' that doesn't even exist, and there is no guarantee the test will pick up a real problem.

More reliable indicators of an increased risk of cervical cancer are a family history of the disease, taking the contraceptive pill or hormone replacement therapy, and smoking.

Other risk factors include a high number of sexual partners, becoming sexually active at an early age, numerous pregnancies, and having genital herpes or genital warts. Symptoms to watch out for are a persistent vaginal discharge and any bleeding in between periods. If none of these risk factors applies to you then your risk of cervical cancer is very low.

Alternative approaches can help reverse cervical dysplasia and lower your risk of cancer

If you smoke, this is probably the incentive you need to give up, as doing so will cut your cancer risk dramatically. And if you are taking the contraceptive pill, it is worth considering another hormone-free form of contraception.

Follow a healthy, balanced diet that excludes sugar and artificial additives and cuts down on dairy produce and red meat (because of hormone residues), salt, coffee and alcohol. Eat plenty of vegetables (especially broccoli and other members of the cabbage family that are high in natural cancer fighters), garlic, oily fish, nuts and seeds.

Nutritional deficiencies also play a major role in the onset of cervical dysplasia and cervical cancer. Most important is vitamin A and its predecessor compound, beta-carotene. Low levels of beta-carotene are linked to a 300 per cent increase in the risk of cervical dysplasia *(Nutr. Cancer 6: 49-57, 1984)*. Take 150,000 to 200,000 IU of beta-carotene a day (you do not need to take vitamin A as well, as your body will convert as much beta-carotene as it needs into vitamin A). Depleted levels of vitamin C have also linked to cervical dysplasia *(Am. J. Ob. Gyn. 151: 978-80, 1985)*. Take 3g a day.

Abnormalities in the cervical cells are often an early sign of folic acid deficiency. *(Am. J. Ob. Gyn. 104: 931-8, 1969)*. In clinical trials, supplementing with folic acid has reversed cervical dysplasia in up to a staggering 100 per cent of cases (*J. Am. Med. Assoc. 226: 1421-4, 1973*). Take 2mg a day of folic acid for the first three months, then cut back to 500mcg a day.

Vitamin B12 should always be taken with folic acid and there is evidence that a B6 deficiency is common in women with cervical cancer too (*Nutr. Cancer 6: 176-80, 1984*). Take 3mg of B12 and 150mg of B6 a day for the first three months, then cut back to one third of the dose.

What to do if your smear test result shows an abnormality

Despite the inaccuracy of many smear tests, it is still important to have them carried out as they can detect cervical cancer and early treatment is crucial. If you receive a negative smear test result your first assumption should be that it is a mistake, so ask to have the test repeated (if possible by a different doctor or clinic). If there is still an abnormality, check whether cells are merely 'atypical', or classed as 'dysplasia'.

For an 'atypical' smear or 'mild' dysplasia, your best course of action may be to wait a further six months and have another test, as many 'mild' abnormalities clear up of their own accord. If you have 'moderate' or 'severe' dysplasia, you could ask for a colposcopy – this is a painless examination of your cervix, which is carried out with a fibre-optic microscope to determine the extent and severity of the problem.

Whether you then have a biopsy or surgery to destroy abnormal cells is, of course, a personal choice. If you do so, it should be because you have weighed the pros and cons and come to an informed decision, not one based on fear.

If you're found to have cervical cancer you may need to have other tests to find out if the cancer has spread. These may include a computed tomography (CT) scan, a magnetic resonance imaging

(MRI) scan or an ultrasound scan. Over the next few years positron emission tomography (PET)-CT scanning will replace these as the best procedure.

Gardasil® is not the 'fairytale cancer vaccine' it's dressed up to be

There are more than 100 subtypes of the human papillomavirus (HPV) and most women who are sexually active will have had the virus at some stage in their life. Usually, the body's natural defences defeat the virus, and most women never even know they had it in the first place.

Exposure to certain strains of HPV induces changes in some cells in the cervix. These affected cells can potentially go on to develop cervical intraepithelial neoplasia (CIN, sometimes called dysplasia or dyskaryosis), and progress into cervical cancer.

Two vaccines have been developed to prevent infection with the human papillomavirus (HPV). These are called Gardasil® and Cervarix®.

Gardasil® protects against four types of HPV:

• 16 and 18 (high-risk for cervical cancer).
• 6 and 11 (low-risk for cervical cancer but causes genital warts).

Cervarix® just protects against HPV types 16 and 18.

Both vaccines are licensed (doctors can prescribe them) in the UK. Gardasil® can be prescribed for women between the ages of nine and 26. Cervarix® can be given to women aged between 10 and 25.

The vaccines don't protect against all types of HPV and women may be infected with more than one type, so it is not guaranteed that they will prevent cervical cancer. It is, however, expected that vaccination will prevent most of the more serious precancerous changes (CIN 2 and 3). Gardasil® is also expected to prevent most genital warts.

However, so far, more than 1,500 Britons have experienced adverse reactions to Cervarix®. While most have included minor complaints such as rashes, swelling on the injection site, pain or allergic reactions; more worrying problems such as seizures and epileptic fits have been reported.

In the US, where Gardasil® is the vaccination of choice, over 11,900 girls and young women have reported adverse events following the jab – including paralysis, coma, seizures and more. The number of deaths reported is currently between 32 and 45, based on different sources. That number may seem statistically low compared to the number of girls that have received it, but if it were your daughter, the statistics wouldn't matter.

As already mentioned, there are more than 100 subtypes of the human papillomavirus. Gardasil® is effective against only four strains. Does this mean we have to wait for 96 more dangerous vaccines to be developed for 'protection' against the rest of these strains? Risking more lives and more adverse effects? Feeding the money-hungry pockets of pharmaceutical giants, whilst there are other effective alternatives available such as screening and smear tests.

The vaccine maker Merck claims there is no link between Gardasil® and serious adverse events and says that the vaccine is usually well tolerated; the most likely side effects include – pain, itching, swelling at the injection site, fever, nausea, and dizziness...

Yet in the US, The National Vaccine Information Center, a private vaccine-safety group, compared Gardasil® adverse events to another vaccine, one also given to young people, but for meningitis. Gardasil® had three times the number of Emergency Room visits – more than 5,000, and reports of side effects were up to 30 times higher with Gardasil®.

While all of this is going on, Merck has asked the American Food and Drug Administration (FDA) to approve it for boys, who can pass on the cancer-causing virus to girls, meaning the number of people getting Gardasil® may soon double.

Treatment options for cervical cancer

If caught at their earliest precancerous stage, abnormal cervical cells can be dealt with simply.

Treatment options for cervical cancer include surgery, radiotherapy and chemotherapy. Sometimes these treatments are used in combination. Your surgeon or oncologist will advise you which treatment is best for you.

Microinvasive disease – This means that the cancer hasn't spread outside your cervix and has not penetrated very far into the cervix. A minor operation to remove the cancer might be all that is needed. You may have one of the following procedures:

- Laser therapy (also known as laser ablation) uses heat to destroy the abnormal cells.
- Cold coagulation, which, despite the name, also uses heat to destroy abnormal cells.
- LLETZ (large-loop excision of the transformation zone) or loop diathermy, uses a heated loop of wire to remove the abnormal areas. The cells aren't destroyed so the tissue can be sent to a laboratory for testing.

If you're older and have completed your family, your surgeon may offer a total hysterectomy (removal of the cervix and womb).

If you have disease that has penetrated further into the cervix you may have a:

- radical hysterectomy (removal of your cervix and womb, nearby tissue and the top of your vagina)
- hysterectomy with lymphadenectomy (removal of the lymph nodes in your pelvis)
- hysterectomy with radiotherapy (a treatment to destroy cancer cells with radiation)

Radical trachelectomy may be an option for some early cancers if you still want to have children. In this procedure your surgeon will remove most of your cervix, but leave enough behind so that it may still be possible for you to have a baby afterwards. There is a slightly higher risk of treatment failure when trachelectomy is used in place of radical hysterectomy.

Invasive disease – If your disease is at a later stage, you may need surgery, radiotherapy and/or chemotherapy.

Surgery – A radical hysterectomy may be performed. Your surgeon will also remove your nearby lymph tissue to see if the cancer has spread.

Radiotherapy – A beam of radiation is targeted on the cancerous cells, which shrinks the tumour. If the cancer has spread beyond your cervix, it's unlikely that surgery alone will be able to treat it and radiotherapy with chemotherapy is the usual treatment. Radiotherapy can also be used after surgery to help reduce the risk of the cancer coming back. Radiotherapy can be given either from outside your body (external beam radiotherapy) or internally (brachytherapy). These treatments are usually given in sequence.

Chemotherapy – Chemotherapy is a treatment to destroy cancer cells with medicines. It's usually given as a series of injections into a vein. Chemotherapy is normally given at the same time as radiotherapy to make the treatment more effective. This is called concomitant chemoradiotherapy. Chemotherapy is sometimes used before radiotherapy or surgery to shrink a tumour. It can also control symptoms if cancer comes back after an initial treatment.

Chapter Nine: Pancreatic Cancer – the 'silent disease'

Your pancreas has two main purposes: 1) it produces the digestive enzymes that break down food; and 2) it's the source of hormones (insulin and glucagon) that are important in controlling the amount of sugar in your blood. There are two types of pancreatic cancer – carcinoma of the pancreas, and, far more rarely, cancer of the cells which make insulin.

Pancreatic cancer develops in about 1 in 10,000 people each year in the UK. Most cases are in people over 60. The symptoms are subtle, so it's rarely diagnosed in the early stages when treatment is most effective. This is how pancreatic cancer came to be known as the 'silent disease'.

Overall, pancreatic cancer has a poor prognosis – it is the fifth most common cause of cancer death in the UK. By the time someone has symptoms, goes to their doctor and is diagnosed, the disease is very often quite advanced.

The most common symptom is abdominal pain, which occurs in approximately 70 per cent of cases. Jaundice is the second most common symptom, occurring in approximately 50 per cent of cases.

In addition, nausea, vomiting, weight loss, changes in bowel habits and the onset of diabetes can all indicate that the disease is present.

If pancreatic cancer is suspected, there are a number of tests your doctor can carry out

One such test involves a physical examination – although it can be very difficult to feel a pancreatic cancer due to its position in the body. Your pancreas is located in your upper abdomen and lies behind your stomach and intestines (guts). The shape of your pancreas is like a tadpole, with a 'head', 'body' and 'tail'. The head section is nearest to your duodenum (the part of the gut just after your stomach).

Blood tests are also carried out, including pancreatic amylase and liver function tests. Confirmatory tests include CT and MRI scans, and ERCP (endoscopic retrograde cholangiopancreatography) or the use of ultrasound. A special type of ultrasound scan, which is done during an endoscopy or telescopic investigation of the intestines, enables doctors to look at your pancreas from deep inside your body. This sort of scan is known as an endoluminal ulatrasound or EUS.

A biopsy operation is the only sure way to complete a diagnosis. This involves taking a tiny tissue sample from the tumour. In some cases, a probe is passed through a small cut into your abdomen to see how far the disease has spread. Occasionally a more serious 'laparotomy' operation is needed – this involves making a larger cut so that the surgeon can look more closely at the organs.

Blood tests may be done to check for general signs of disease such as anaemia, as well as chemical markers in the blood which provide clues about certain types of cancer. These tests, and a small operation to look inside the abdomen if necessary, help the doctors to work out how far it has advanced and decide whether an operation to remove the cancer might help. They also help to give an idea of prognosis or long-term outlook.

The lowdown on the treatment options available

Unfortunately, only about 15 per cent of people diagnosed with pancreatic cancer survive past a year, and only three per cent live for more than five years after diagnosis. Those people whose cancer is caught early have a better prognosis, as do those who are generally fitter. Some less common types of pancreatic cancer also have better survival rates.

Treatment options that may be considered include surgery, chemotherapy and radiotherapy. A combination of therapies can either cure the cancer if caught early, or, if not, improve quality of life and reduce pain.

Surgery – If the cancer is at an early stage, then there is a modest chance that surgery can be curative. An early stage means a small tumour which is confined to within the pancreas and has not spread to the lymph nodes or other areas of your body.

If the tumour is in the head of the pancreas then an operation to remove the head of the pancreas may be an option. This is a long and involved operation as the surrounding structures such as the duodenum, stomach, and bile duct need to be rearranged once the head of the pancreas is removed.

If the tumour is in the body or tail of the pancreas then removal of the affected section of the pancreas is sometimes an option.

The reason why the chance of cure is only modest is because in a number of cases thought to be at an early stage, some cells have already spread to other parts of the body but are not yet detectable by scans or other staging tests. In time they grow into secondary tumours.

If the cancer is at a later stage, then surgery is not an option to cure the disease. Some surgical techniques may still be able to help ease symptoms. For example, it may be possible to ease jaundice caused by a blocked bile duct. A 'bypass' procedure may be used, or a stent may be inserted into the bile duct. A stent is a small rigid tube made of plastic or metal which aims to keep a duct or channel open. It is usually inserted by instruments attached to an endoscope.

Chemotherapy – Chemotherapy involves the use of anti-cancer drugs which kill cancer cells and help stop them from multiplying. When chemotherapy is used in addition to surgery it is known as 'adjuvant chemotherapy'. For example, following surgery you may be given a course of chemotherapy. This aims to kill any cancer cells which may have spread away from the primary tumour.

Radiotherapy – Radiotherapy is a treatment which uses high energy beams of radiation which are focused on cancerous tissue. This kills cancer cells, or stops cancer cells from multiplying. Radiotherapy is not commonly used to treat pancreatic cancer.

Research uncovers simple ways to prevent pancreatic cancer

According to Dr Halcyon Skinner, Ph.D, a Northwestern University researcher in the US: "Because there is no effective screening for pancreatic cancer, identifying controllable risk factors for the disease is essential for developing strategies that can prevent cancer."

The two most prominent controllable risk factors are obesity and cigarette smoking, both of which raise your risk of developing the cancer. In fact, it is estimated that 1 in 5 pancreatic cancers are caused by cigarette smoking.

In addition to quitting smoking and losing any excess weight, Dr Skinner led a study that shows how supplementing with one particular vitamin may reduce pancreatic cancer risk by a surprisingly significant degree *(Cancer Epidemiology, Biomarkers & Prevention, Vol. 15, No. 9, September 2006)*.

Enter vitamin D…

Looking for dietary or environmental factors that might affect pancreatic cancer risk, Dr Skinner and his team analyzed data from two long-term population studies that followed the medical conditions and dietary habits of more than 122,000 subjects. About 75,000 subjects were women, and most of the subjects were over the age of 40.

Three key results stood out:

- Subjects who took supplements that supplied at least 400 IU of vitamin D per day (the recommended daily allowance) lowered their risk of pancreatic cancer by 43 per cent.
- Those who took vitamin D supplements that supplied less than 150 IU of the vitamin per day lowered their risk by 22 per cent.
- Those who took more than 400 IU per day did not lower their risk by any more than 43 per cent.

The best source of vitamin D is sunlight. When your skin is exposed to ultraviolet light, your body responds by manufacturing vitamin D. Unfortunately, the amount of sun needed to develop vitamin D is only available in the UK during the summer months.

Another promising research finding in the fight against pancreatic cancer

While you're upping your vitamin D intake, there's another dietary choice that may help lower pancreatic cancer risk.

Canadian researchers investigated a possible link between pancreatic cancer and dietary intake of carotenoids; organic plant pigments that have been shown to help control inflammation. Subjects included 462 patients diagnosed with pancreatic cancer, and more than 4,700 healthy people selected from eight Canadian provinces.

Researchers found that beta-carotene and total carotenoid intake was associated with a significantly reduced risk of pancreatic cancer among non-smoking subjects. But the most striking result concerned the carotenoid lycopene. Those who had the highest lycopene intake reduced their pancreatic cancer risk by more than 30 per cent, compared to subjects with the lowest intake.

The richest dietary source of lycopene is tomatoes, and absorbency of this important antioxidant is increased when tomatoes are served warm with a source of fat, such as cheese or meat.

Studies have shown that lycopene may also offer protection against breast cancer, prostate cancer and heart disease.

Pancreatic cancer study update: How fish oil can reduce symptoms of cachexia

A new study conducted in the UK shows that fish oil could eventually become a standard of cancer care in addressing cachexia. Researchers at the Royal Infirmary in Edinburgh created a study to examine the effects of omega-3 fatty acid supplements on weight, lean body mass, dietary intake, and general quality of life in advanced pancreatic cancer patients with symptoms of cachexia.

People with cancer and other chronic diseases often experience cachexia – a general loss of vitality characterised by poor appetite, weight loss, decomposition of muscle and depression. These symptoms also compromise the immune system and make the body susceptible to other illnesses.

Two hundred patients were divided into two groups: 95 received a daily high-calorie/high-protein supplement, enriched with vitamins C and E, and about 2g of omega-3 fatty acids; and 105 received a similar supplement that didn't include the additional vitamins or fatty acids.

At the beginning of the study, subjects were losing an average of approximately 7lbs pounds per month. But over the eight-week period of the study, subjects in both groups stopped losing weight. When researchers conducted a specific analysis of dose-response relationships, they found that the omega-3 group showed significantly higher rate of weight gain, as well as increased lean body mass compared to the other group. Furthermore, weight gain was associated with improved quality of life only in the omega-3 group.

Exactly how the enriched supplement created greater benefits over the other supplement isn't known. Nor is it clear that this sort of supplement might have the same effect on patients suffering from cachexia due to other types of cancers or diseases. Nevertheless, the Edinburgh team concluded that supplements enriched with omega-3 fatty acids from fish oils apparently have positive effects on cachexia symptoms, especially those of weight loss and diminished quality of life.

Although dietary sources like walnuts and flaxseed deliver good amounts of omega-3, only fish contain both eicosapentaenoic acid (EPA) and docohexaenoic acid (DHA). When combined, these two fatty acids have been shown to help prevent Alzheimer's disease, arthritis, influenza, hyperactivity, and even some forms of cancer, in addition to the benefits mentioned above. The highest concentration of omega-3 fatty acids is found in oily fish such as tuna, swordfish and salmon.

Chapter Ten: Ovarian Cancer

Nearly 5,500 women are diagnosed with cancer of the ovary every year in the UK and it is the fifth most common cancer in women. There are several different types of ovarian cancer, but by far the most common – accounting for 90 per cent of cases – is epithelial ovarian cancer, or cancer of the surface layers of the ovary.

The rest are mostly 'germ cell' tumours. These are a group of cancers of the egg-making cells of the ovary. Other rarer cancers can also affect the ovary, for example, sarcomas.

Could you be at risk?

As with most cancers, the risk of developing ovarian cancer increases with age. Most cases are in women who are past their menopause. A family history of cancer is one of the most important risk factors for ovarian cancer. About 1 in 10 ovarian cancers, 10 per cent, are caused by an inherited faulty gene. Other possible risk factors include infertility, using HRT, being overweight or tall, having endometriosis and using talcum powder.

Screening is currently only offered to those at high risk, for example, because of a family history. In particular you may be at increased risk and offered screening if you have close relatives (sibling, parent or daughter) who've had one of the following types of cancer – breast, colon, prostate or endometrial (lining of the womb). In addition, women who have previously suffered from breast cancer are twice as likely to get ovarian cancer in the future.

You may want to have a look at Macmillan's OPERA tool: http://opera.macmillan.org.uk. This online risk assessment program has been designed to give information about your hereditary risk based on your personal and family history of breast and ovarian cancer.

Like pancreatic cancer, ovarian cancer is often well advanced before any symptoms arise. Many women with early stage cancer of the ovary don't report any symptoms at all. Early symptoms can include pain in the lower abdomen or side, and/or a bloated, full feeling in the abdomen. If you experience any of these symptoms it's important you see your doctor as the success rate for treatment of ovarian cancer is very high when the disease is caught in the early stages.

Later stage disease can cause symptoms from the tumour growing in the pelvis. This can cause irregular periods, lower tummy (abdominal) pain, back pain, passing urine more often than usual, constipation, pain during sex, or a swollen abdomen.

Advanced ovarian cancer can cause even more symptoms because the cancer has spread into the abdomen or elsewhere in the body. These can include a loss of appetite, feeling or being sick, constipation, tiredness, shortness of breath, or a noticeable swelling of the abdomen.

Diagnosing the disease

To help make a diagnosis your doctor will carry out a full pelvic examination, feeling for the presence of an abnormal lump. However, it's only as a tumour grows and spreads that the symptoms become clearer and the problem easier to diagnose. If your GP can feel a lump in your tummy, or has other cause for concern, you should have an urgent ultrasound scan. Your GP may also request some additional tests, including:

- Blood tests.
- A consultant gynaecologist will go on to perform a laporoscopy, which is where keyhole surgery is used to look at the female internal organs, including the ovaries, fallopian tubes and uterus, with the patient unconscious under a general anaesthetic. A biopsy, which means a small piece of tissue is taken from the ovary, will also be done. If any problems are suspected with your

digestive system, an endoscopy will be arranged, to look at your stomach, or a colonoscopy, to look at your lower bowel. If there is a lot of fluid within the abdomen due to ovarian cancer, the consultant will do an abdominal tap, which allows some of the fluid to be drawn off under a local anaesthetic. The fluid can then be examined under a microscope for cancer cells, or drained off to make the patient more comfortable.

- Chest X-ray to check for spread of the cancer into your lungs.
- CT or MRI scan – also to check for any possible spread elsewhere in your body.

Ovarian cancer – treatment and recovery

Surgery is almost always the first treatment a woman with ovarian cancer undergoes. This normally involves the removal of the ovaries, the womb and the fallopian tubes, which link the two. Usually both ovaries are removed, unless the patient has only a slow growing cancer in one, and wants her fertility to be preserved.

The surgeon cannot always be sure that all the cancerous cells have been removed, so chemotherapy is almost always given as well, to kill any which remain in the body.

However, treatment will depend on your general health, the type of cancer, how far it has spread and the severity or grade of the cancer. Many cases will continue to respond to multiple courses of chemotherapy. Chemotherapy can be given after surgery, or beforehand in selected cases.

A landmark study funded by the National Cancer Institute in the US recently revealed that a promising drug used in the treatment of bowel, breast and lung cancer could also help to extend the lives of women with advanced ovarian tumours. The study revealed that taking bevacizumab (Avastin), in combination with standard chemotherapy, can offer women an extra four to six months of life without their disease getting worse.

Radiotherapy is used occasionally to kill cancer cells in the pelvic area. Ongoing trials are studying hormone treatments and biological therapies.

Many factors increase or reduce a woman's chance of beating ovarian cancer. The main one is the spread of the disease – if caught early, as with many cancers, it's much more treatable, particularly if only one part of one ovary is involved. If the cancer involves a whole ovary, both ovaries, or has spread to involve other tissues, the chances of a cure are reduced.

Also important is the type of ovarian cancer – some affect the cells which line the womb, whereas some affect the cells which produce eggs. Both have different cure rates. Overall the quality of life of ovarian cancer patients has improved considerably over the last 10 years.

High folate intake can help ward off ovarian cancer

A new study shows how the intake of one important nutrient might significantly reduce the risk of ovarian cancer. Studies have shown that in addition to lowering homocysteine levels and reducing the risk of stroke, folate may also help prevent breast and colorectal cancer. Knowing that this water-soluble vitamin could be a key to the prevention of some cancers, researchers at the Karolinska Institute in Stockholm, Sweden, designed a study to examine how folate intake might be associated with ovarian cancer.

Using records from the Swedish Mammography Cohort, researchers examined data on a group of more than 61,000 women ranging in age from 38 to 76 years old. None of the women were diagnosed with cancer at the outset of the study. On average, the dietary and medical records of the women were followed for about 15 years.

The researchers found that when the women with the highest folate intake were compared to the women with the lowest intake, those in the higher group had a slightly reduced risk of developing ovarian cancer. More striking, however, was the fact that women who had folate-rich diets and who also drank at least two or more alcoholic beverages each week were 74 per cent less likely to develop ovarian cancer.

Obviously, two drinks a week is a fairly moderate intake of alcohol. But this is one of those cases where more is not better, because excessive alcohol consumption can create a folate deficiency. Other factors that can lead to low folate levels include: smoking, oral contraceptives, high intake of aspirin, general malnourishment, and certain drugs such as the chemotherapy drug methotrexate.

The Karolinska Institute researchers noted that their findings were based on dietary questionnaires, so further studies would be required to determine if supplements of folate might be just as effective as dietary sources of the vitamin.

Fortunately, dietary sources of folate are easy to come by. Citrus fruits, tomatoes, leafy green vegetables, avocados, bananas, asparagus, whole grains, and pinto, navy and kidney beans are all good sources of folate.

Supplements of folate are available as natural (folate) or synthetic (folic acid). The daily recommended intake (DRI) of folate is 400mcg, but for those trying to lower homocysteine levels, at least twice that amount is necessary. Pregnant or nursing women are also urged to take a folate supplement of 400mcg per day to prevent a deficiency of the vitamin. In the Karolinska Institute study, those in the higher-intake group were getting a minimum of about 200mcg per day.

Some additional details need to be considered when taking folate supplements. You should be aware that a high intake of folate can mask a vitamin B12 deficiency in older people. However, a vitamin

B12 deficiency can be easily avoided by eating meat, fish and eggs, or by taking B12 supplements.

Health Sciences Institute panellist Dr Allan Spreen, recommends folate supplements of 1.6mg (1,600mcg) per day, and as much as 5mg for those who want to address cardiovascular problems. Dr Spreen points out that, "Folate isn't effective in low doses except in a limited percentage of cases." And to avoid a deficiency of B12, he recommends 1mg (1,000mcg) per day in sublingual form (dissolved under the tongue).

In addition, Dr Spreen also suggests that to get the most out of folate, 100mg per day of B6 is also necessary, as well as 400-500mg of magnesium per day (to make the B6 more effective). If you take a good quality multivitamin, you're probably already getting a good foundation of these nutrients. But when addressing specific health concerns, Dr Spreen recommends that you beef up the B vitamins and folate to reach these totals.

Good news for tea lovers

Australian researchers have found that drinking one cup of tea a day could help reduce the risk of ovarian cancer. Those drinking two cups a day or more see a slightly greater benefit, with their cancer risk reduced by about 12 to 13 per cent. Green tea is known to have beneficial effects, but research, published in the journal *Cancer Causes and Control*, shows that black tea – the kind most widely consumed in Britain – may be almost as effective.

Ovarian cancer protection from gingko

In a study conducted at the Brigham and Womens Hospital, in the US, researchers examined the use of herbs in treating ovarian cancers. The researchers found that women who took herbal gingko biloba had a 60 per cent lower risk of this type of cancer.

The US scientists looked at over 1,200 women, half of whom had ovarian cancer. After six months, the women who took herbal gingko biloba had a 60 per cent lower risk for ovarian cancer.

The women in the study commonly used gingko, echinacea, St John's wort, ginseng and chondroitin. But analysis showed that only gingko was linked to ovarian cancer prevention.

Women who had non-mucinous ovarian cancers had an even more pronounced preventative effect, with the data showing a reduced risk of 65 to 70 per cent.

The scientists discovered that the most active components that contributed to gingko's protective effects were ginkgolides A and B.

Lead researcher, Dr Bin Ye stated that, in the future, these findings could potentially offer a new strategy for ovarian cancer prevention and therapy, using the active forms of ginkgolides.

Get up and get moving

There have been several studies focusing on exercise benefits for breast and colon cancers, but few on ovarian cancer... until now.

A recent study found that regular moderate exercise and work-related physical activity may reduce the risk of ovarian cancer.

Canadian researchers looked at over 2,500 women, 442 who were diagnosed with ovarian cancer. The scientists had their patients fill out questionnaires asking details about physical activity. The results showed a lower risk of ovarian cancer with high levels of moderate exercise, but not for vigorous activity. Women with jobs that required moderate or strenuous activity also experienced a reduction in ovarian cancer risk compared with those who worked in sedentary occupations.

Chapter Eleven: Lung Cancer

Lung cancer is the most commonly diagnosed cancer in the world. In the UK, it's the second most-frequently occurring cancer, accounting for one in seven new cases.

Anyone can develop lung cancer, but people who smoke (or used to smoke) are most at risk – nine out of 10 cases are caused by the effects of tobacco smoking. The risk increases with the total number of cigarettes you smoke.

If you stop smoking, the risk gets less over time and after about 15 years the chances of developing the disease are similar to that of someone who has never smoked. Researchers are trying to find out if there is a genetic reason why only some smokers get lung cancer, but as yet there is no clear answer to this question.

Lung cancer has always been more common in men, particularly those aged over 40. However, as fewer men smoke now rates have fallen. Meanwhile, lung cancer rates increased among women until the 1980s as more took up smoking. Although rates among women have stabilised, the disease now claims more lives than breast cancer.

Passive smoking over a long period of time can occasionally cause lung cancer too. Some rare types of lung cancer aren't related to smoking. Mesothelioma, which affects the covering of the lung (the pleura), for example, is almost always caused by exposure to asbestos. Other causes include exposure to certain chemicals and substances in the workplace, such as uranium, chromium and nickel.

There are several different types of lung cancer, which are generally divided into:

- Non-small cell lung cancer (NSCLC); this includes 'squamous' cell cancers and 'adenocarcinoma'

- Small cell lung cancer (SCLC)

How to recognise the symptoms that can spell lung cancer

The key symptom of lung cancer is a persistent cough that gradually gets worse.

In addition, if you have any of the following symptoms you must have them checked out by your doctor (but bear in mind that they can occur in many other conditions):

- A persistent cough or change in the nature of a longstanding cough
- Shortness of breath
- Coughing up blood-stained phlegm (sputum); blood is a warning sign that always needs urgent investigation
- Persistent chest pain – a dull ache or sharp pain when you cough or take a deep breath, However, pain usually only occurs if the tumour reaches the edge of your lung
- Loss of appetite and weight
- A drop in your ability to exercise and general fatigue

In a few cases where the tumour has spread outside the lungs, the first symptom may not come from the chest at all, for example:

- liver jaundice (when the colour of your skin or eyes becomes yellow)
- bone pain or fracture
- skin lump
- nerve or brain damage affecting walking, talking, behaviour or memory

---

How is lung cancer diagnosed?

By the time symptoms appear, the tumour can nearly always be seen on a chest X-ray. If lung cancer seems likely then you will be seen by a hospital chest specialist within two weeks.

The specialist may need to carry out a biopsy – whereby a sample of tissue is taken to be analysed. There are different ways of taking a biopsy:

- If your tumour is near the middle of your lung, the chest specialist will use a bronchoscope. This is a very small telescope, and the test is done under sedation, so you won't feel anything.
- If your tumour is near the edge of your lung, an X-ray specialist (radiologist) will pass a needle into your chest, using a local anaesthetic to numb the area.
- Occasionally it is necessary to perform a minor operation under general anaesthetic to be sure of getting a good specimen.

You may also be advised to have a CT scan. This provides information about:

- The lung tumour in more detail.
- Exactly where and how big it is.
- Whether the cancer has spread outside your chest.
- Which sort of biopsy would be most helpful.

A CT scan involves lying on a cushioned table which moves through a large metal hoop. You will be given an injection in your hand, and the machine will take pictures of your chest and stomach area. The whole procedure only takes a few minutes.

A new diagnostic tool identifies the earliest stages of lung cancer with a non-invasive procedure…

Every breath you take has a unique chemical signature that can reveal the health of your lungs. That prompted US researchers at the Cleveland Clinic to examine a method that reads the signature of an individual's exhaled breath to determine the presence of lung cancer in its earliest stages – a breakthrough that could significantly lower lung cancer mortality rates.

In the medical journal *Thorax*, the Cleveland researchers note that volatile organic compounds (VOCs) are created when metabolic changes occur within cancer cells. The Cleveland team tested a technique that uses a small array of chemically sensitive sensors that detect VOC patterns unique to cancer. The sensors are small spots on a disposable cartridge. The spots change colour if specific VOCs are present in exhaled breath.

Study profile:

- Of 143 subjects recruited for the trial, 122 had different types of respiratory disease.
- Nearly 50 subjects had been diagnosed with small cell lung cancer.
- Researchers examined sensor results from 70 per cent of the subjects in order to establish a predictive model.
- With this model, the remaining 30 per cent were tested.
- About three out of four cases of lung cancer were successfully predicted.
- Results were not affected by the varying stages of cancer.

Further trials of this promising technique are needed to confirm its effectiveness. And hopefully those trials are underway, given that the only common breath testing techniques for lung cancer (mass spectrometry and gas chromatography) are very expensive and require such specific expertise that early stages of lung cancer are often missed.

Treatment options available

Treatment of lung cancer depends on the type of tumour, its location and how far it has spread, as well as the person's general health. A process known as 'staging' is used in each case to assess these factors and recommend appropriate treatment.

Unfortunately, non-small cell lung cancer (NSCLC) is hard to cure, and in many cases, the treatment given will be to prolong life as far as possible and to relieve symptoms. Small cell lung cancer (SCLC) is different; in particular, it has a tendency to spread to distant parts of the body at a relatively early stage. Chemotherapy and/or radiotherapy are usually more effective in treating this type of lung cancer because it has usually spread to more than one place by the time it's diagnosed and is less likely to be cured by surgery.

Surgery – A small number of people with lung cancer can be offered an operation – usually when the tumour is away from the centre of the chest and there's little or no spread (typically in NSCLC).

Removing lung cancer is a major operation, and it will take you a number of weeks to recover fully. A small part of the lung may be removed, or the entire lung. You can breathe normally with only one lung. However, if you had breathing difficulties before the operation you may be more breathless afterwards. Breathing tests will be carried out to help you and your doctor decide on the best course of action.

Sometimes surgery is more successful if you have chemotherapy either before or after your operation.

Radiotherapy – This uses high-energy X-rays to destroy cancer cells. It is arranged by a specialist called a 'clinical oncologist'. You might be offered either:

- A long course of treatment ('radical radiotherapy'). This aims to cure the cancer if the cancer is small, but an operation is not possible. It means daily trips to the hospital for treatment over several weeks. This therapy can cause temporary side effects like tiredness, dry throat or problems with swallowing.

- A short course of treatment ('palliative radiotherapy'). This aims to improve symptoms such as cough, bleeding, pain or breathlessness. This only involves between one and five visits to the hospital and generally causes few side effects.

New hope for advanced lung cancer patients too sick for chemotherapy

The latest research findings have revealed how a drug called erlotinib or Tarceva (which works by interfering with how cancer cells multiply) can extend life for women with advanced lung cancer and reduce their chances of dying by a quarter.

They offer hope for those with advanced lung cancer who are too sick to undergo chemotherapy. According to Cancer Research UK,

---

which ran the trial, almost half of the 39,750 lung cancer patients in the UK fall into the category of being too ill for chemotherapy.

The study involved 670 men and women with advanced NSCLC, of whom more than half were over the age of 77. The researchers revealed that 15 per cent of women were alive and had no progression of their cancer 12 months after taking the drug, compared with only 5 per cent of those taking a placebo.

Dr Siow Ming Lee, trial leader and senior lecturer at the University College London Cancer Institute, said: "These results are a real step forward in the search for an effective treatment for patients with advanced lung cancer. We are not yet sure why it was most effective in women but this is positive news for this large group who have few other treatment options. Erlotinib should be recommended for women with non-small cell lung cancer who are unsuitable for first-line chemotherapy."

The drug is currently licensed in the UK to be used as a second-line treatment after chemotherapy.

Chemotherapy – This involves using drugs to treat cancer. It has the advantage that the drugs go straight into your bloodstream where they can attack the cancer cells wherever they are, including outside the lung. But since chemotherapy also affects normal cells, temporary side effects are common.

Treatment involves having a drip and receiving drugs by injection and tablets, usually as an out-patient. You would usually have two courses ('cycles'), and then have another CT scan to see how you are responding. If chemotherapy is working you may be given four to six cycles in total, every three weeks.

Symptom control – If your cancer is found to be at an advanced stage or is making you feel unwell, you might decide with your doctors that none of the treatments described above is right for you.

You might benefit from a palliative approach. This focuses on the symptoms you are experiencing, such as cough, breathlessness, poor appetite or weakness, and using medicines or other treatments to control them. The purpose is to improve the quality of your life so that you feel as well as possible.

Your specialist might recommend referring you to a palliative care team who can visit you and your family at home. Some of these teams are linked to a local hospice, and can provide lots of additional help and support to you during your illness.

How simple dietary changes can reduce your risk of lung cancer

According to the latest research findings, high blood levels of vitamin B6 and the amino acid methionine appear to offer a protective effect against lung cancer in smokers and non-smokers alike *(Journal of the American Medical Association, June 16, 2010; vol 303: pp 2377-2385).*

Lead researcher Dr Paul Brennan, of the International Agency for Research on Cancer in Lyon, France, says: "We found that vitamin B6 and methionine are strongly associated with reducing lung cancer risk in people who never smoked, those who quit, and current smokers."

Dr Brennan and his fellow researchers evaluated levels of B6 and methionine in blood samples from participants in the large European Prospective Investigation into Cancer and Nutrition (EPIC) study, which enrolled more than 519,000 participants from 10 European countries between 1992 and 2000.

His team zeroed in on 899 lung cancer cases and compared them to a group of 1,770 healthy comparison-group participants, matched to the lung cancer patients by country, sex, date of birth, and when the blood was collected.

They classified the participants into four groups, depending on blood levels of vitamin B6, which helps the body break down protein, maintains red blood cells, and performs other bodily functions; and methionine, which is involved in B vitamin metabolism.

After accounting for smoking, the researchers found that the higher the levels of vitamin B6 and methionine, the lower the lung cancer risk: People in the highest group for vitamin B6 levels had a 56 per cent reduced lung cancer risk, compared to those in the lowest group. Those with the highest methionine levels had a 48 per cent reduced lung cancer risk.

Commenting on the findings the researchers said: "Given their involvement in maintaining DNA integrity and gene expression, these nutrients have a potentially important role in inhibiting cancer development, and offer the possibility of modifying cancer risk through dietary changes."

Vitamin B6 is found in beans, grains, meat, poultry, fish, and some fruits (bananas are a rich source of the vitamin) and vegetables. Methionine is found in animal protein, some nuts, and vegetable seeds.

Another, unrelated study involving diet and lung cancer has revealed that pomegranate extracts can inhibit the growth and replication of human lung cancer cells *(Carcinogenesis 2007; 28(1):163-73).*

Chapter Twelve:
The natural anti-cancer therapies showing real promise against the disease

As seen in the previous chapters focusing on specific types of cancer, there is a wealth of evidence to support the use of a growing number of natural remedies and complementary treatments in the fight against cancer.

Whilst natural remedies should not be thought of as an alternative to conventional treatment for cancer, they can play an important role when used, with your doctor's prior approval, alongside conventional treatments. It is extremely important that cancer patients inform their doctor before self-medicating with any of the supplements listed, and their progress should be carefully monitored by their doctor.

There is evidence that some natural remedies are able to prevent the disease and even help combat existing cases from spreading (metastasising) to other organs. In many cases they help to rebuild the body's natural immunity and strengthen its own ability to destroy cancer cells.

Consider the following: One of the reasons modern medicine continues to fail in its war against cancer is due to how the disease is viewed. Conventional therapies focus on the end result of the disease – tumours. Yet the tumours are manifestations of a more generalised process.

Cancer researcher Mauris L Emeka puts it as follows: "Think of the malignant tumour for what it is: it's an indication that a process has gone wrong. In other words, the tumour is a visible symptom telling us that the body's metabolism is not working properly."

So, it is possible that cancer is not simply a genetic disease...

something that a growing body of research now strongly supports. Instead it is a disease in which normal cell division is disturbed by external factors such as chemicals, radiation, toxins, stress and the modern diet and lifestyle.

If this is the case, what are the alternatives for treating cancer, instead of simply cutting away or radiating the symptoms? The following are some of the most promising natural therapies available. What is striking about them all is that they work from the basic principle that cancer starts with toxins in the body and that that is where the prevention and healing starts.

• Vitamin C: A valuable addition to any anti-cancer arsenal

The idea that vitamin C, also known as ascorbic acid, could be used to treat cancer was advanced in the 1970s by American scientist Linus Pauling. He is one of a small number of individuals who received a Nobel Prize more than once.

The foundation of his theory (and the way it is applied today) can be explained in the following simple terms: Vitamin C is a major water-soluble antioxidant. When injected in high doses it can also act as a pro-oxidant. These are agents that generate free radicals as well as produce hydrogen peroxide, which has tumour-killing abilities.

The vitamin C will then oxidise tissues, which is what chemotherapy does. But there is a difference: whilst having anti-cancer effects, the vitamin C also preserves normal, healthy cells – which chemotherapy doesn't always do.

When attacking cancer with vitamin C, absorption is the key issue. For instance, 10g of IVC prompts blood levels of the vitamin that are many times higher than that achieved with the same amount of the vitamin when taken orally.

Vitamin C at pro-oxidant levels can only be achieved with an intravenous infusion. The most common procedure is to use 75g of vitamin C, in sterile water, with a number of minerals, particularly magnesium, zinc, chromium, selenium, B12 and some B vitamins.

The patient is infused over 2.5 hours daily for three weeks. Vitamin C levels are tested at the end of the infusion course and if it is sufficiently high then some significant tumour kill has occurred. This process may have to be repeated depending on the individual results of the infusion course.

In a laboratory study, researchers at the National Institute of Diabetes & Digestive & Kidney Diseases (NIDDK) in the United States exposed normal cells and 10 types of cancer cells to a dose of vitamin C that could be easily reached using intravenous vitamin IVC.

In five of the cancer cell types, about half of the cells were either killed or apoptosis (cell suicide) occurred. Vitamin C exposure also halted most of the growth of surviving cancer cells. The normal cells were completely unaffected.

The *Canadian Medical Association Journal (CMAJ)* has published details on three IVC/cancer case studies:

Case One: A 51-year-old woman with kidney tumours refused conventional treatment. Instead, she received 65g of IVC twice each week. She also used other supplements such as N-acetylcysteine and niacinamide. After 10 months of IVC, her tumours were gone. Her cancer remained in complete remission for four years, at which point she was diagnosed with lung cancer (she had been a long-time smoker). She began IVC therapy again, but it wasn't successful in treating the lung cancer. She died one year later.

Case Two: A 49-year-old man with a bladder tumour and multiple satellite tumours, declined chemotherapy and radiation. He began an

IVC regimen of 30g twice each week for three months, followed by 30g once every two months for four years. During those four years he sometimes took more frequent treatments. Nine years later, the man is in good health with no recurrence or spreading of the cancer. Other supplements used in this patient's regimen include flax oil, selenium and alpha lipoic acid.

The authors of the *CMAJ* article note that standard treatment for muscle invasive bladder cancer is complete or partial bladder removal. When treated without surgery, this cancer type almost invariably spreads to other organs within a short period.

Case Three: After receiving six weeks of radiation therapy to treat lymphoma, a 66-year-old woman declined chemotherapy and began receiving 15g of IVC twice each week for two months. She continued with a less frequent IVC regime for another 19 months. Ten years later the patient is in good health and cancer-free. In addition to vitamin C, the patient also took a variety of supplements that included beta-carotene, CoQ10, N-acetylcysteine and a multiple vitamin (*Intravenously Administered Vitamin C as Cancer Therapy: Three Cases Canadian Medical Association Journal, Vol. 174, No. 7, 3/8/06*).

It appears that IVC not only successfully addresses some cancers, but for some patients it also relieves the debilitating side effects of chemotherapy. Here's what a lady called Donna wrote on the *Health Sciences Institute* health forum:

"My best friend has been on the chemo routine for cancer (non-Hodgkin's lymphoma); she has had five chemos every six weeks. She is also getting 50 grams of vitamin C intravenously three times a week. She has had no side effects from either, in fact she goes shopping after the chemo, and leads a normal life.

During the Christmas holidays she discovered that it's the vitamin C that is preventing side effects from the chemo, as she wasn't able to get the treatments. After seven days without C she was in pain all over and had sores inside her mouth. When she went back after 10 days for a treatment of vitamin C she was feeling much better just during the drip of vitamin C. The next day she was completely fine again."

Should antioxidant supplements be avoided during chemotherapy?

In a nutshell, here's how the controversy goes: Cytotoxic therapies (such as certain chemo and radiation therapies) create free radicals that are believed to help prompt the death of cancer cells. In the late 90s, a few researchers theorised that free radical-fighting antioxidant supplements might make the therapies less successful.

Some have even gone so far as to suggest that patients treated with cytotoxic therapies should avoid antioxidant-rich foods. This would basically cut all beneficial fruits and vegetables out of an ailing person's diet!

Dan Labriola was one of the first researchers to theorise this antioxidant/cytotoxic conflict. In 1999, Dr Labriola reported in the journal *Oncology* that patients who took antioxidant supplements had poorer responses to some cytotoxic therapies compared to patients who didn't use supplements.

Dr Labriola suddenly found himself in no-man's land. As a naturopathic physician he was not treated with respect by the mainstream, and with his anti-antioxidant position he was roundly denounced by the alternative medicine community.

But the response from the alternative crowd wasn't a knee-jerk reaction. There was already quite a bit of evidence that antioxidants can be helpful in fighting cancer, even when used with cytotoxic therapies.

Research shows that antioxidants can extend cancer patients' lives

Ralph W Moss is one of the foremost authorities on alternative cancer treatments. In 2000, Dr Moss published a book titled *Antioxidants Against Cancer*, in which he outlined the ways antioxidants actually enhance the effectiveness of cytotoxic treatments while minimising their side effects.

And Dr Moss' position is backed up by considerable research. For instance, a Life Extension Foundation (LEF) article stated that Dr Charles Simone – a medical and radiation oncologist who helped establish the Office of Alternative Medicine for the National Institutes of Health in the US – has cited more than 350 studies that demonstrate how antioxidants have extended cancer patients' lifespans while improving their quality of life.

The LEF article also featured a pioneer of nutritional healing and dietary supplement treatments, Dr Abram Hoffer. Dr Hoffer has used mega doses of vitamin C to successfully treat well over 1,000 cancer patients, most of whom were also receiving chemotherapy.

At a 2001 biomedical symposium, Dr Moss gave a speech that included this comment: "We can reassure patients that the overwhelming mass of data accumulated so far supports the concurrent use of chemotherapy with dietary antioxidants."

As for supplementary antioxidants, *Health Sciences Institute* panellist Dr Allan Spreen offers this outline of a cancer treatment regimen that includes a familiar antioxidant: "Most alternative doctors, whether they use chemo, modified chemo (a powerful technique called Insulin Potentiated Therapy, or IPT), or no chemo, nearly ALL utilise vitamin C in VERY high doses. The key is using it intravenously on non-chemo days, as it is used up very quickly in times of stress (cancer would more than qualify). Chemo acts fairly quickly, and the vitamin C tends to protect normal cells more than cancer cells, which it helps to kill in many cases."

And Dr Spreen adds: "I'd have to see a TON of highly definitive evidence before I'd stop taking supplements with my cancer treatment."

- **Antineoplaston therapy helps trigger the death of cancer cells**

Antineoplastons are components of the body's natural biochemical defence system that help control cancer without destroying normal cells. Chemically, the antineoplastons include peptides, amino acid derivatives and organic acids. They occur naturally in blood and urine and they are reproduced synthetically for medicinal use.

Antineoplastons act as molecular switches, which turn off life processes in abnormal cells and force them to die through apoptosis (programmed death of a cell). While they trigger the death of cancer cells, they do not inhibit normal cell growth. Antineoplastons 'turn on' tumour suppressor genes and 'turn off' oncogenes (genes participating in the onset and development of cancer) restoring the proper balance in gene expression.

Antineoplaston therapy is given intravenously or orally, depending on the stage and development of the cancer. In one study 74 per cent of children with low-grade brain-tumours saw a marked improvement in their condition whilst receiving the therapy. In the same study 91 per cent of patients with colon cancer were still alive after five years compared to just 39 per cent of those who received the conventional chemotherapy.

- **Discover how your health could benefit from cutting-edge enzyme therapy**

Researchers are fast discovering that life expectancy and quality of life is directly proportional to the efficiency of your body's enzyme system. Indeed, many leading scientists and doctors now believe that low enzyme levels are the primary cause of nearly all diseases, including cancer, and are also responsible for accelerating the ageing process.

It's not difficult to see why this might be the case when you consider that we are made up of a staggering 70 million cells and that our bodies perform 200 million chemical processes daily – from the production of energy to the removal of harmful toxins and cancer-causing free radicals from your body.

Every single one of these 200 million processes, which also include helping your immune system fight infections, is controlled and regulated by an enzyme produced by the body specifically for that individual process.

Digestive enzymes, many of which are made in the pancreas, break down food and help with the absorption of nutrients into the blood. Metabolic enzymes build new cells and repair damaged ones in the blood, tissues and organs.

Enzyme therapy is based on the premise that a cancer cell is coated with a protein lining to protect it against the body's normal immune defences. Certain enzymes can dissolve this cell lining, thereby allowing the body's white blood cells to destroy the cancer cells.

Pancreatic enzymes were reportedly first used to treat cancer in 1902 by John Beard, a Scottish scientist. German researchers later used enzyme therapy to treat patients with multiple sclerosis, cancer, and viral infections.

Enzyme levels can quickly become depleted

Your enzyme levels can decrease as a result of numerous factors including the consumption of processed foods. This is because the high levels of artificial chemicals and preservatives they contain places an increased demand on your body, and many important enzymes are used up in the process of neutralizing their harmful effects.

In a similar way, stress, lack of exercise, and even ageing itself cause an increased requirement for enzymes. Eventually, if stores become depleted over time then you become vulnerable to chronic diseases like cancer, heart disease and dementia.

The first typical symptoms of low enzyme levels – which is a common but not widely recognised problem – include fatigue, loss of energy, dizziness, allergies, digestive disorders and skin problems *(Pharmacogenomics. 2006 Apr; 7(3):365-73).*

Fortunately a ground-breaking new product called Regulat® has just been launched that aims to ensure you have optimal amounts of enzymes in your body that function at peak capacity. It is particularly beneficial if you have been experiencing the symptoms of low enzyme levels.

Special manufacturing process enhances Regulat's® healing potential

Regulat® contains bio-accessible, active enzymes from a combination of different organic fruits, vegetables and nuts that have all been specially selected for the wide range of health-giving properties they possess.

The active enzymes from these foods are obtained in liquid form through a process called cascade fermentation *(Appl Microbiol Biotechnol. 2006 Aug; [Epub ahead of print]).* This process involves the use of activating chemicals such as biologically fortified water and lactic acid, which break the enzymes down to ensure that they will be properly absorbed through the intestinal villi and into the bloodstream where they can get to work.

Regulat® also contains other beneficial bioactive compounds such as micro-organisms ('friendly' bacteria) and micronutrients (minerals and amino acids) *(J Biosci Bioeng. 2006; 101(3): 274-6).*

By delivering an additional supply of health-giving enzymes, your own levels remain intact

All of the ingredients in the preparation work on the same principle, in that they facilitate the body's various chemical processes by providing the enzymes needed for these reactions to take place. This avoids the need for your body to use up its own limited supply of enzymes. The ingredients in Regulat® also work together to activate existing enzymes within your body, which then help your cells work more effectively. These ingredients include:

Celery – is a powerhouse of essential oils, which help fight a variety of infections in the digestive tract including the mouth, stomach and bowel. These essential oils also have beneficial actions on the nervous system and help ease anxiety. And, as scientists have just discovered, a chemical called luteolin, which is present in celery, can reduce the risk of cancer and even prevent existing cancerous cells from spreading *(Am J Physiol Gastrointest Liver Physiol. 2006 Aug; [Epub ahead of print])*.

Figs have been included in the formula because they contain enzymes that promote digestion and aid weight loss. They also possess powerful antibacterial properties that help accelerate the healing of wounds. In addition, research has shown that they can improve mood, counteract nervousness, combat fatigue and sluggishness, boost concentration and ease symptoms associated with menstruation *(Forum Nutr. 2006; 59: 154-70)*.

Walnuts are a rich source of essential fatty acids (also known as the 'good' fats) such as alpha-linoleic acid. Researchers have found that essential fatty acids can help lower high cholesterol and combat heart disease *(Am J Cardiol. 2006; 98 (4 Suppl 1): 3-18)*.

Saffron is a spice that has been used for thousands of years, both as an ingredient in many Indian dishes and also as a medicine – particularly for relieving hot flushes associated with the menopause.

In addition, recent research shows that it helps improve memory and cognitive skills *(Behav Brain Res. 2006 Oct 2; 173(1): 112-5).*

Artichokes. The main ingredient in artichokes is cynarin – a natural plant chemical that promotes the production of bile acids, thereby aiding digestion. Cynarin is also an antioxidant that helps protect the liver against harmful toxins *(Am J Clin Nutr. 2006; 84(1): 95-135).*

Regulat® contains so many beneficial ingredients that it is difficult to go into them all here in depth. To summarise: the formula also contains peas – a rich source of the mineral magnesium, which is needed for healthy nerves and muscles. Millet has been added for its high content of quality proteins, silicic acid and lecithin together with several minerals such as iron, copper and manganese – all of which boost hair and nail growth among other health benefits.

Sprouts contain flavonoids, vegetable protein and vitamins that are necessary for the optimal functioning of your liver and kidneys. The final ingredient in Regulat® is coconut – it contains both calcium (that helps keep osteoporosis at bay) and fatty acids that are needed for healthy circulation and brain function.

What to take for best results

The recommended dose for Regulat® is 10ml taken twice a day.

IMPORTANT: You should not take Regulat® if you suffer from a nut allergy as the product contains walnuts.

• Ozone therapy delivers supercharged oxygen to your body

Ozone – which is supercharged oxygen – has important medical benefits, including anti-cancer ones, when administered at the correct therapeutic levels. Oxygen therapy is based on the fact that poor oxygenation of the blood produces conditions that are especially conducive to the growth of bacteria, viruses, fungi and cancer cells.

Dr Otto Warburg, twice Nobel Laureate, is credited with proving that cancer cells cannot thrive in an oxygenated environment.

"Cancer, above all diseases, has countless secondary causes, but there is only one prime cause: anaerobic respiration."

In other words, lack of oxygen in the body at a cellular level makes it more conducive for cancer cells to grow. Dr Warburg stated that when there is insufficient oxygen for normal aerobic respiration, cells go into "fermentation mode". Cells grow out of control, becoming cancerous. Further research proved that this can be reversed by saturating the cells with oxygen.

Oxygenating the blood is the main aim of ozone therapy. Flooding cells with oxygen may retard the growth of cancer cells or even help to return them to normal. One of ozone's primary effects is to increase blood oxygenation by stimulating the production of ATP (adenosine triphosphate), which activates red blood cells to transport more oxygen to tissues. By encouraging the production of white blood cells that help your body fight infection, ozone is a potent immune system stimulant.

Ozone can be medically applied to the body in a number of ways (mainly by the use of an ozone generator that produces ozone by electrical discharge). The ozone is then used in various ways:

Infusing Blood: This involves drawing blood from the patient and then infusing it with ozone. Once the patient's blood is infused with O3 it is then returned to the body through a drip. This treatment is repeated on a daily basis.

Ozonated Water: Ozonated water is created by bubbling O3 through purified water. It can then be used in various ways in order to oxygenate the tissues. Some doctors directly inject ozonated water into tumours.

Other ways of ozonating the blood include enemas, direct application of ozonated olive oil and bathing in ozonated steam. Air tight body bags are also used in order to surround part or all of the body in ozone.

These therapies are still at the stage of evaluation by the medical profession as a whole. However, they have been legalised in some countries and some parts of the US.

Hydrogen Peroxide: Hydrogen peroxide (often used as a disinfectant) is also used in oxygen therapy. One of its special qualities is its ready ability to decompose into water and oxygen.

It is involved in all of the essential processes of life, including the immune system – it is the body's first line of defence against viruses, bacteria, parasites and yeasts, as it carries an extra molecule of oxygen that is released to attack these invaders, which are killed by oxygen. Hydrogen peroxide is produced by granulocytes, the white blood cells that fight infection.

The theory behind hydrogen peroxide therapy is that it is used to supplement the body's own supply of oxygen. In a laboratory study, hydrogen peroxide was found to have anti-tumour effects on cells (*J Exp Med, 1981; 154: 1539-53*).

Researchers have revealed that, when combined with radiation therapy, it can enhance the effect and spare normal tissue from the effects of radiation. In a study, 190 patients with advanced cancer (considered beyond the help of conventional medicine) were selected – in fact, less than a tenth of the patients were expected to survive for more than a year. After a combination of hydrogen peroxide therapy and radiation, 77 per cent were alive after a year, two-thirds after two years, nearly a half after three years and one-quarter after five years.

The best results occurred in sufferers with cervix, bladder, head or neck cancers *(Am J Surg, 1964; 108: 621-9)*.

Hydrogen peroxide is either taken orally or it is injected into the bloodstream in a diluted form. Again it must be stressed that this therapy is still being evaluated and must only be carried out under professional medical guidance.

Hyperbaric Oxygen Therapy (HBOT) involves the breathing of pure oxygen while in a sealed chamber. The air pressure is raised up to three times higher than normal air pressure. Under these conditions, your lungs can gather up to three times more oxygen than would be possible breathing pure oxygen at normal air pressure.

The increased oxygen dissolves in your blood during hyperbaric oxygen therapy, and circulates throughout your body. Oxygen-rich blood stimulates your body to release substances called growth factors and stem cells, which promote healing.

It is generally used for treating decompression sickness, carbon monoxide poisoning, stroke and brain damage, but has been used by some clinics for treating cancer. It has also been found to be useful as an additional method for the prevention and treatment of osteoradionecrosis (bone damage caused by radiation therapy).

Caution: It is vital that you seek the care of an experienced ozone therapy practitioner as inhalation of the gas can damage your lungs.

• Gerson Therapy boosts the health of your liver and helps rid your body of harmful toxins

The Gerson Therapy is a powerful, natural treatment that boosts your body's own immune system to heal cancer, arthritis, heart disease, allergies, and many other degenerative diseases.

One aspect of the Gerson Therapy that sets it apart from most other treatment methods is its all-encompassing nature. An abundance of nutrients from 13 fresh, organic juices and food are consumed every day, providing your body with a super dose of enzymes, minerals and nutrients. These substances then break down diseased tissue in the body, while enemas aid in eliminating the lifelong build-up of toxins from the liver.

One of the major aspects of the therapy is to restore liver integrity – to enable the body to heal. The liver has many different functions vital to the healing process of the body.

Organic juices are used because they are easily absorbed. In people with compromised immune function the digestive system is usually under-functioning. The nutrients from juices are easily absorbed into the bloodstream in 15-30 minutes. Organic food is used because pesticides add to the toxic burden. The main aim of this therapy is to clear overall toxicities from the cells.

One cancer sufferer to benefit from the Gerson Therapy is Michael Gearin-Tosh…

Michael Gearin-Tosh's story of alternative cancer treatment

Michael Gearin-Tosh's book titled *Living Proof: A Medical Mutiny*, about alternative health care for cancer is incredibly moving because it offers insightful advice as well as tremendous hope for anyone who may be faced with a cancer diagnosis…

In 1994, at the age of 54, Michael Gearin-Tosh, a don of English literature at Oxford University, was diagnosed with multiple myeloma, a cancer of the bone marrow, considered to be treatable but not curable. Less than 3 per cent of multiple myeloma patients survive 10 years. When diagnosed, he was told that with aggressive chemotherapy he might live two years. Against all odds, Gearin-Tosh went on to live for 11 years.

On one level, Gearin-Tosh's story is about the world of challenges that every cancer patient experiences. The aspect that sets his story apart from so many others is the course of treatment he chose. After being told by one specialist that treating his cancer with a dietary regimen would be 'useless', and after consultations with several doctors, a good deal of personal research, and discussions with family and friends, Gearin-Tosh chose to forego chemo, opting instead for less abrasive alternative treatments.

The road to therapy

During the first weeks after his diagnosis, Gearin-Tosh researched different treatments on his own while weighing the advice of friends. During this conflicted time (made no easier by the anaemia associated with his disease) he consulted several doctors, some of who were impersonal in their manner and vague when answering his questions.

They insisted that immediate chemotherapy was the only reasonable way to go. What Gearin-Tosh found lacking was a rational support for chemotherapy. He wondered: If chemo is not a cure, then what's the point? When pressed to explain the merits of chemo, all they could offer was further insistence that it was his only option.

But the book is in no way a diatribe against the medical profession. One doctor, (a consultant, retired from practice), became a reliable guide without ever pushing the patient in a direction he didn't want to go. Another doctor helped advise him on a wide variety of options, both conventional and alternative.

Finally, two months after his diagnosis, just as he was about to reluctantly begin chemotherapy, Gearin-Tosh made a breakthrough in his research of treatments when he learned about a New York City physician – Dr Nicholas Gonzalez – who had successfully treated many cancer patients with detoxification, vitamin supplements, and a strict diet of vegetable juices.

Although he didn't become a patient of Dr Gonzalez, Gearin-Tosh cancelled his chemotherapy and proceeded with a dietary regimen (based on the Max Gerson cancer therapy) in combination with high doses of vitamin supplements (following the guidelines of Linus Pauling and Dr Abram Hoffer). He also practised visualisation techniques involving special breathing exercises, took coffee and castor oil enemas (to stimulate detoxification in the liver), and visited an acupuncturist on a regular basis.

A living part

One of the most striking things about this book is the way Gearin-Tosh tells his story. He saves it from being a grim tale by frequently interjecting moments of gentle humour and interesting characters (such as a houseguest, a captain in the Russian Army, who Gearin-Tosh discovers one morning cooking breakfast and drinking champagne at 6am).

More importantly, Gearin-Tosh never preaches. He doesn't urge other cancer patients to embrace any particular therapies. He doesn't suggest, for instance, that acupuncture or coffee enemas or drinking fresh carrot juice will save the lives of all cancer patients. And he doesn't even condemn chemotherapy, noting that certain doctors have developed specialised chemo techniques combined with bone marrow transplants that have helped make chemotherapy more effective in treating multiple myeloma.

Instead, in what Gearin-Tosh calls the core of his argument, he encourages cancer patients to be open-minded, questioning, and to trust their instincts. He believes that the ideal goal is to become an involved, 'living part' of any therapy that's chosen. But with the thoughtfulness of someone who's been there, he tempers this advice with the phrase, 'if you feel you can'.

Nutrition, nutrition, nutrition

The book concludes with an eloquent, peer-reviewed case history of the patient, written by Carmen Wheatley, a former student of Gearin-Tosh's, and one of his most dedicated supporters throughout his treatment period. Dr Wheatley (a doctor of philosophy) concludes the history with a statement by Dr Jeffrey Bland, a biochemist who simply states that every cancer therapy should include nutritional consultation as a standard of care – otherwise this should be considered 'malpractice by omission'.

- **New research has revealed a link between low levels of vitamin D and cancer**

Dr Cedric Garland and his colleagues at the University of California in the US, believe they may have found a new model of cancer development. They suggest that cancer, rather than commencing with genetic mutations within cells, is initially caused by a reduction in the ability of cells to stick together *(Ann Epidemiol 2009, 3 April [Epub ahead of print])*.

This discovery may not seem to have much to do with everyday life. Not until you read that inadequate vitamin D can result in a loss of stickiness between cells, as well as a loss of differentiation, which causes cells to revert to a stem cell-like state. In plain English this means that if you are deficient in vitamin D, you may be at greater risk of developing cancer.

This new model is one of progressive phases of cancer development. It starts with the loss of cell stickiness, which leads to a loss of communication between cells. In healthy tissue, cells are constantly 'talking' to one another and this reinforces their identity, for instance as being part of a liver, or a thyroid gland, or a breast.

When the communication between cells breaks down, they appear to suffer an identity crisis – they no longer know what they are supposed to be. In this situation, cells undergo genetic mutations and the most rapidly reproducing cells become dominant. These non-specific, fast-growing cells are the ones that become cancers.

Dr Garland's cancer model opens up new avenues for preventing and improving the success of cancer treatment: "Vitamin D may halt the first stage of the cancer process by re-establishing intercellular junctions in malignancies having an intact vitamin D receptor," he says.

Dr Garland has carried out several studies concerning the relationship between low sunlight exposure and vitamin D levels with an increased risk of breast, colorectal, ovarian and kidney cancers. In fact, more than 200 epidemiological surveys have associated certain cancers with reduced vitamin D status.

New, independent research, published in the *Journal of Clinical Oncology*, shows that women diagnosed with breast cancer have a better chance of beating it if their vitamin D levels are adequate (*J Clin Oncol 2009, 18 May [Epub ahead of print]*).

Researchers at the University of California in San Diego, looked at more than 120,000 women in the UK and the US. Blood tests were carried out on a sample of the group with breast cancer, and on a sample without.

In a few cases, where the women had unusually high levels of vitamin D, they showed a 50 per cent reduced risk of breast cancer. In cases of more modestly raised levels of vitamin D, the risk was still reduced by 10 per cent.

To supplement, take 1,000 to 2,000 IU of vitamin D daily and try to get half an hour's sun exposure on your face and arms on sunny days, without using sunscreen. If the sun is very strong, though, do your sunbathing early or late in the day.

- **Tocotrienols could reduce DNA damage that leads to cancer**

Several studies show that tocotrienols – the less studied from of vitamin E – may have a significant effect on cancer cells. In one study, tocotrienols inhibited the growth of human breast cancer cells by 50 per cent, whereas alpha-tocopherol had no such effect *(Lipids, vol. 30, pp. 1139-1143, 1995)*.

Another study, investigating liver cancer, found that "tocotrienol supplementation (reduced) the impact of carcinogens in rats" *(Nutrition, vol. 9, pp. 229-232, 1993)*. Tocotrienols also exhibit "strong activity against tumour production", while tocopherols were found to be ineffective *(International Journal of Cancer, vol. 57, pp. 529-531, 1994)*.

It's too bad that so much of the recent research on vitamin E has studied alpha-tocopherol only. Because tocotrienols are far more biologically active, many researchers theorize that they will provide all of the documented benefits of alpha-tocopherol – only more so.

New research suggests that tocotrienols may reduce DNA damage (considered an important trigger in cancer development) by about 50 per cent.

Researchers from Universiti Kebangsaan Malaysia and tocotrienol-supplier, Golden Hope Bioganic, found that daily supplementation with a tocotrienol-rich supplement (Tri E Tocotrienol) showed greater effects in older subjects – a sub-population with higher rates of DNA damage.

Lead researcher Siok-Fong Chin said: "The effect of Tri E Tocotrienol is more obvious in older age, possibly reflecting a greater need for supplementation or a greater profound effect due to the larger amount of damage present."

This randomised, double-blind placebo-controlled study involved 64 subjects aged 37 to 78, who were assigned to receive daily supplements of tocotrienol-rich vitamin E (160 mg/d, Tri E Tocotrienol, Golden Hope Bioganic) for six months. The supplement contained all four tocotrienols and alpha-Toc in a ratio of 74:26 per cent, respectively.

The researchers found that white blood cells from patients receiving the tocotrienol-rich supplement had significantly less DNA damage after three and six months of supplementation than those in the placebo group.

Significant reductions were also observed for urinary levels of 8-hydroxy-2-deoxyguanosine (8-OHdG) – a marker for oxidative stress – in the supplementation group, relative to placebo.

Supplementation with the tocotrienol-rich vitamin E also reduced the frequency of sister chromatid exchange (SCE) – an exchange of genetic information between sister chromatids that may be related to tumours, particularly in the older participants (over 50).

The researchers believe that this mechanism of protection is related to oxidative stress and the quenching of reactive oxygen species by vitamin E. The free radical theory of ageing (FRTA) places free radicals at the front of causes for deterioration of physiologic function as people get older.

Commenting on the findings the researchers said: "The results obtained suggested that supplementation with palm oil Tri E Tocotrienol reduced the level of DNA damage in healthy subjects, with a more pronounced effect observed in older adults. These observations may indicate a possible relation between the molecular mechanisms involved in the formation and repair of DNA breaks with Tri E Tocotrienol supplementation."

Therapeutic levels can't be obtained from food sources alone

Both tocopherols and tocotrienols are available from your diet. Corn and wheat (staples of the Western diet) are rich in tocopherols, while mainstays of the Eastern diet – most notably rice bran and palm oil – contain tocotrienols.

Over the years, several rice bran 'miracle cures' have come and gone in the marketplace. The benefits attributed to these formulations are most likely due to their tocotrienol content. A higher consumption of rice is no doubt partially responsible for the lower levels of heart disease and cancer observed in Asian cultures.

However, it would be virtually impossible to achieve therapeutic levels of vitamin E through food sources alone. To ingest 200 IUs of vitamin E, you would have to consume 10 cups of almonds, which are among one of the richest food sources of vitamin E. Obviously, supplements are the best choice.

If there's a downside to tocotrienols, it's this one practical matter: In supplement form, full spectrum tocotrienols tend to be more expensive than full spectrum tocopherols. But so far the research would indicate that the extra expense is worth it.

• Essiac: Myth or Miracle?

Two years before she died in 1978 at the age of 90, a Canadian nurse called Rene Caisse, decided at last to reveal the formula of an ancient North American Indian remedy which she had guarded all her life.

The Remedy, called Essiac (Caisse spelt backwards), was a bitter brown mixture of burdock root, sheep sorrel, Turkish rhubarb root and slippery elm bark. She claimed it was the key to long-lasting immune system health and protection against a host of diseases, including cancer.

Anecdotal reports indicate Essiac's powerful anti-cancer properties

Rene was introduced to the Remedy in 1922 while working in a hospital in Ontario. Bathing an elderly patient, she noticed a shrunken scar on the woman's breast. According to the woman this marked the site of a tumour which, 20 years earlier, had nearly killed her. She explained how she had discovered a lump while living in a mining camp in a remote region of northern Canada, which was later diagnosed as breast cancer. Terrified of surgery, she confided in a friend who called on the services of an Indian medicine man from the Ojibwa tribe, who gave her a herbal tea to drink. Within months, the woman told Rene, the lump had gone. Understandably, Rene was sceptical but, intrigued, she took down the formula from the woman.

When Rene's aunt subsequently developed breast cancer, Rene gave her the herbal brew with the approval of her aunt's physician, Dr R Fisher. Both Rene and Dr Fisher were impressed with the effect of the remedy in helping to fight the cancer, and her aunt lived for 21 years following the diagnosis.

Rene and Dr Fisher worked to refine the formulation, and from the mid-1920s onwards Rene treated thousands of people who flocked to her clinic in Ontario, as news of Essiac spread. She charged no fee and asked only for voluntary contributions to cover her costs.

The doctors who became convinced of the power of Essiac

Rene's work was opposed by many orthodox cancer specialists but she did attract the attention and support of several eminent medical practitioners, including Dr Charles Brusch of the prestigious Brusch Medical Center, and former physician to President John F Kennedy. Dr Brusch wrote that: "Essiac has merit in the treatment of cancer" and in a sworn affidavit made on 6 April 1990, he testified that: "I endorse this therapy even today."

After word of Rene's impressive results spread, Dr John Wolder, at Northwestern University Medical School in Chicago, arranged, in 1937, for her to treat 30 terminal cancer patients under the direction of five doctors. After one and a half years of Essiac therapy, the Chicago doctors concluded that Essiac prolonged life, shrank tumours and relieved pain.

In addition, Dr Frederick Banting, the world-famous co-discoverer of insulin, believed that Essiac was also capable of stimulating the pancreas in diabetics into normal functioning. (However, the research necessary to confirm this observation has yet to be carried out.)

A bittersweet legacy

Rene rejected large sums of money throughout her life to make Essiac available commercially, desperate to prevent the formula falling into the wrong hands. She feared drug companies and unscrupulous quacks would charge vast sums for it, thus depriving the people who really needed it to safeguard their health.

Despite her misgivings, Rene knew she must pass on the secret of Essiac before she died. Unfortunately, her legacy has failed to benefit mankind in the way she hoped. Essiac has been the subject of bitter squabbles and in-fighting between various parties who claim to have Rene's 'own formula', and the medical establishment who ridicule the claims being made for the remedy.

Consequently, the herbal mixture that was once taken by tens of thousands of people who, according to anecdotal records, reported amazing, healthful benefits, has remained one of the best kept secrets of underground medicine.

The potent herbs in Essaic have many therapeutic benefits

Herbalists believe that the synergistic interaction of ingredients contributes to the overall therapeutic effect of a herbal remedy. However, there is good evidence that at least two of the herbs in Essiac are extremely potent in their own right.

Burdock root is the key active ingredient in Essiac. In 1966, two Hungarian scientists reported "considerable anti-tumour activity" in a purified fraction of burdock. And in 1984, Japanese scientists at Nagoya University discovered in burdock a new type of desmutagen – that is a substance uniquely capable of reducing cell mutation which can lead to cancer.

Scientists at the Memorial Sloan-Kettering Hospital in New York tested sheep sorrel, between 1973 and 1976. On 10 June 1975, Dr Chester Stock, a Sloan-Kettering vice-president, concluded that there was: "test data in two experiments indicating some regressions in sarcoma 180 (a type of tumour) of mice treated with Essiac".

When taken as a nutritional herbal mixture, Essiac appears to boost the functioning of the immune system in its ability to deal with potentially danagerous rogue cells.

References:

1. Miners, S.E. Essiac, new hope for cancer sufferers. Health Consciousness Magazine 15(2): 1-5, 1994.
2. Bohlen, C. Naming a saint isn't so simple. The New York Times, Section 4, September 14, 1997, p.1
3. Snow, S., personal communications by tape recording, mail, and teleFAX.
4. Thomas, R. The Essiac Report. (Los Angeles: The Alternative Treatment Information Network, 1993), pp. 17&18.
5. Caisse, R.M. I Was "Canada's Cancer Nurse" (New Action Products: Buffalo, New York, 1996).
6. Snow, S. The Essence of Essiac. (Port Carling, Ontario: Sheila Snow, 1996), pp. 116 & 117.
7. Ibid.
8. Walters, R. Options: The Alternative Cancer Therapy Book. (Garden City Park, New York: Avery Publishing Group, Inc., 1993), pp. 112 & 113.
9. Glum, G.L. Calling of an Angel. (Los Angeles, California: Silent Walker Publishing, 1988).
10. Op. cit. Thomas, R., The Essiac Report, Appendix, Exhibit Four.
11. Lewis, J. and Berger, E.R. New Guidelines for Surviving Prostate Cancer. (Westbury, New York: Health Education Literary Publisher, 1997), p.362.
12. Fink, J.M. Third Opinion, second edition (Garden City Park, New York: Avery Publishing Group, Inc., 1992), p. 94.
13. Diamond, W. J.; Cowden, W.L.; Goldberg, B. An Alternative Medicine Definitive Guide to Cancer (Tiburon, California: Future Medicine Publishing, Inc.. 1997), p. 36.
14. Journal of the American Holistic Veterinary Medical Association 12(4):29-30, Nov. 1994 - Jan. 1995.
15. Townsend Letter for Doctors & Patients.
16. The Holistic Health Network

- **How a substance found in broccoli could revolutionise the way we tackle cancer**

The fact that broccoli promotes good health is hardly ground-breaking news. It's a great source of nutrition, providing us with vitamins C and E, iron and folic acid, as well as bioflavonoids, such as beta-carotene, which is known to have a powerful anti-cancer action.

Broccoli's cancer-fighting properties have been well documented over the years, particularly its ability to protect against breast, prostate and colon cancer *(JAMA. 286: 2975-2977; Cancer Epidemiol, Biomark. Prev. 9: 795-804; Cancer Epidemiol. Biomark. Prev.9: 477-485; National Cancer Institute analysis 1987; Sun D. 2010. University of Michigan Comprehensive Cancer Centre study, Clinical Cancer Research Journal).*

As mentioned on page 116, it contains a compound called indole-3-carbinol (I3C) which stimulates the conversion of oestrone, the 'bad' form of oestrogen that promotes breast cancer, into an inactive form called 2-hydroxyoestrone *(Breakspear Medical Bulletin, Summer 2002).*

In the 1990s, Dr Paul Talalay – Director of the Laboratory for Molecular Pharmacology at Johns Hopkins University School of Medicine in Baltimore, in the US – discovered that broccoli is the most potent source of a naturally occurring compound called sulforaphane glucosinolate (SGS) and, most importantly, SGS's precursor, glucoraphanin.

Glucoraphanin has caused a great deal of excitement in the scientific community for its ability to strengthen the body's natural defences against disease, particularly cancer. It helps your defence enzymes to work to their maximum efficiency to protect cells against harmful oxidants, DNA damage and radiation.

This antioxidant-booster effect lasts considerably longer than that of other well-known antioxidants, such as vitamins C and E, which only work over a period of a few hours after ingestion. By contrast, glucoraphanin goes on targeting cancer-causing free radicals and rendering them harmless, up to 72 hours after ingestion.

Thanks to the research team at Johns Hopkins you can now take full advantage of glucoraphanin's cancer-protective powers

So, to benefit surely all you need to do is include more broccoli in your diet, right? Unfortunately, it's not quite as simple as that.

While broccoli is an excellent source of glucoraphanin, one of the problems, up until recently, has been that its levels can vary greatly depending on whether the broccoli is fresh or frozen, how old it is and how it has been stored. As a result it is almost impossible to determine how much glucoraphanin the broccoli you're purchasing at your local supermarket or greengrocers contains.

Continuing research by scientists at the Johns Hopkins University School of Medicine has revealed that the seeds of broccoli contain up to 100 times the levels of glucoraphanin found in the corresponding amount of fresh broccoli.

This exciting discovery led to the development of Comvita® Broccoli Extract, which has just been launched in the UK. It contains a standardised extract of New Zealand-grown broccoli seeds and captures the same amount of glucoraphanin per two capsules, which would be found in approximately 100g (half an average head) of fresh broccoli.

Dr Talalay believes the current focus of cancer research is short-sighted

Comvita's brand-new Broccoli Extract is backed by 15 years of scientific research into the disease-prevention qualities of vegetables carried out by renowned medical scientist and researcher Dr Paul Talalay.

Dr Talalay is a respected pioneer in the field of chemo-protective research and has completed extensive research into broccoli *(Cancer Epidemiology, Biomarkers and Prevention, Vol 7, 1091-1100, December 1998)*. As already mentioned, it was Dr Talalay's 1992 discovery of SGS and glucoraphanin in broccoli that led to this vegetable being the subject of such intensive study.

He believes that it is carcinogenesis (the processes that lead to cancer) that is the disease we should be most concerned about – rather than the cancers themselves. He subscribes to the view that the focus on curing advanced disease has blinded cancer researchers to the possibilities of cancer prevention; we tend to be stuck in the idea that people with cancer are healthy until a doctor tells them that they've got a tumour.

According to Dr Talalay: "Many cells in the body are constantly moving toward malignancy, but fortunately most fail. But carcinogenesis goes largely unnoticed. The number, the location, the state, and the fate of cells moving towards malignancy is mostly unknown. But carcinogenesis is a protracted, multi-stage process, providing many opportunities for intervention. This intervention can take the form of stopping, postponing or even reversing the development of cancer."

"Glucoraphanin is a compound that recharges your protective antioxidant defence enzymes, giving them the power to keep working. This is especially important, as a reduced defence-enzyme level can lead to many chronic diseases," he says.

Unlike other antioxidants, glucoraphanin kick-starts the body's own defence mechanism. It triggers an antioxidant 'cascade' which helps to neutralise dangerous free radicals and interferes with carcinogenic processes *(Cancer Epidemiol Biomarkers Prev 2005; 14 (11))*. Not only has SGS been shown to block the development of cancer, but evidence is steadily mounting that glucoraphanin can help recharge the body's defences against many diseases *(PLOS One July 2008, Volum e3, Issue 7 e2568; Clinical Immunology (2009) 130, 244-251; PNAS October 30, vol 104, 44, 17,500-17,505).*

What to take for best results

The recommended dosage for Comvita® Broccoli Extract is two capsules a day, taken with food.

Pregnant or lactating women should not take this product without first consulting with their healthcare practitioner.

- **How the pulp and rind of citrus fruits have the ability to slow or even halt the spread of cancer**

Lots of research is emerging on modified citrus pectin's (MCP) anti-cancer abilities. It has a unique ability to help prevent cancer cells from spreading – or metastasising – to other parts of the body.

It is demonstrating positive results against some of the most common – and deadly – kinds of cancer, like prostate, breast, colon and lung.

MCP comes from the pulp and rinds of citrus fruits, like oranges and grapefruits, that have been modified so that they produce shorter sugar chains. These shorter sugar chains are more readily absorbed through the intestinal tract and into your bloodstream, where they are able to perform some incredible actions – particularly against cancer cells.

Targeting cancer's means of growth

The shorter sugar chains, or glycans, in modified citrus fruit, are critical to cellular communication. They bind to molecules on cell surfaces called carbohydrate-binding proteins (CBPs) or lectins and pass along all sorts of information. In this case, the sugar chains in MCP seem to target one very specific lectin called galectin-3 that plays a big role in cancer development.

Studies have repeatedly shown elevated levels of galectin-3 in cancerous tissues as compared to healthy tissues. The galectin-3 cancer link has been found in many forms of cancer, including thyroid cancer *(Am J Pathol 1995; 147(3): 815-822; Cancer 1999; 85(11): 2475-2484)*, gastric cancer *(J Comp Pathol 2001; 124(2-3): 216-218)*, pituitary cancer *(Cancer Res 2003; 63(9): 2251-2255)*, breast cancer *(J Natl Cancer Inst 2002;94(24):1854-1862)*, and colorectal cancer *(Prostate Cancer and Prostatic Diseases 2003; 6: 301-304)*.

Galectin-3 also plays a role in a variety of biological functions related to cancer, including tumour cell adhesion and metastasis (spread of the disease) *(Cancer Res 2003; 63(23): 8302-8311)*. Scientists think that galectin-3 accomplishes all of this in two different ways, each utilising one end of its protein molecule structure.

One end, called the C-terminal end, binds carbohydrate molecules on other cells, allowing cancer cells to adhere to each other and to healthy cells. This process allows cancer to spread, or metastasise. The opposite end of the galectin-3 molecule is called the N-terminal. When a specific amino acid called serine binds to the galectin-3 molecule in a certain position on the N-terminal end, it triggers a series of biochemical reactions that protect the cancer cell from apoptosis (death).

Scientists believe this is a two-pronged defence: The galectin-3 kills off immune system cells that are attempting to attack the cancer cells, and it also forms a protective barrier around the cancer cells, shielding them from the effects of anti-cancer drugs and treatments like chemotherapy or radiation *(Cancer Res 2001; 61(12): 4851-4857; Cancer Res 2003; 63(23): 8302-8311)*.

So what does all of this have to do with some grapefruit pulp? MCP's sugar molecules block the protein's ability to bind to carbohydrates on other cancer cells and on healthy tissues by binding to the galectin-3 carbohydrate receptor sites at the C-terminal end themselves. With their binding sites all clogged up, cancer cells can't clump together and can't spread by adhering to other areas.

MCP slows the development of tumours and even kills cancer cells

There have been several significant animal and laboratory studies demonstrating MCP's potential to stop or slow metastases and even kill cancer cells. In one study, mice were fed MCP in their drinking water and then injected with human breast cancer cells or human colon cancer cells. In all cases, MCP effectively inhibited tumour growth, spontaneous metastasis and angiogenesis, the process by which cells develop new blood vessels.

In the breast cancer portion of the study, the tumour volume in mice treated with MCP was less than a third of that of untreated mice. And none of the MCP-treated mice developed lung metastases, while 66 per cent of the untreated mice had tumours on their lungs at the end of the study.

The researchers found similar results in the mice injected with colon cancer cells. The primary tumours of MCP-treated mice were half the size of those in untreated mice. All of the untreated mice developed metastases in the lymph nodes, and 60 per cent developed metastases in the liver. But only 25 per cent of the MCP-treated mice developed cancer in the lymph nodes and none showed signs of cancer in the liver (*J Natl Cancer Inst 2002; 94(24): 1854-1862*).

As far back as 1995, scientists saw similar results in rats injected with human prostate cancer cells and treated with MCP. Nearly all of the untreated rats (15 out of 16) developed lung metastases in 30 days, compared to only 50 per cent of the MCP treated rats (seven out of 14). More than half of the untreated rats also developed lymph node tumours, compared to only 13 per cent of the MCP treated rats *(J Natl Cancer Inst 1995; 87(5): 348-355).*

The results seen in these studies rival the effects of many prescription cancer drugs. But what makes MCP even better is that it doesn't appear to have any dangerous side effects or interactions. Fewer than 5 per cent of people who take MCP report some flatulence or loose stools, due to its soluble fibre content. This can usually be managed by reducing the dose and slowly working back up to the recommended level. But compared to the toxic side effects of most conventional cancer treatments, these problems are very minor.

What to take for best results

It's important to use modified citrus pectin (MCP) – not just regular citrus pectin – to obtain these results; studies have shown that only MCP has the ability to inhibit cancer cell adhesion and galectin-3 activity *(Glycoconj J 1994; 11(6): 527-532).* In fact, nearly all of the research on MCP's effects has been conducted with the same formula: PectaSol®, developed by Dr Isaac Eliaz in the US.

PectaSol® is available in capsules or in powder form; and according to Dr Eliaz most people prefer the powder form because the recommended daily dosage is quite high. To achieve the recommended dose of 14.4g per day you'd have to take six capsules three times a day. You can achieve the same dosage by dissolving 5g of powder in water or juice three times a day.

If you're fighting cancer, talk to your doctor about adding modified citrus pectin to your treatment plan. It may help your body respond better to the treatments you're already undergoing. Or it may just give your body the extra boost it needs to help fight the disease on its own. Either way, it's a valuable addition to any anti-cancer arsenal.

- ## How a trace mineral is showing some truly 'miraculous' results against cancer

Your body contains several 'trace minerals' which, despite being present in minute quantities as their name suggests, are indispensable not only for good health but also for your very existence.

A deficiency in any of these minerals can cause a wide-range of symptoms, which would greatly compromise your overall well-being, such as fatigue, loss of energy, insomnia and an increased susceptibility to various diseases including cancer.

One of the most important of these trace minerals is germanium. A mineral which is not only found in your body but is also present in ginseng, aloe vera, comfrey, and many foods – including garlic, shiitake mushrooms, green leafy vegetables, tuna and oysters.

One of the main functions of germanium is to increase the use of oxygen by your body's tissues, which stimulates your cells to produce energy *(Zhonguan Yu Fang 1994, 28(6): 372-374)*. This makes it an important immune system booster and it is producing some truly remarkable results in the treatment of cancer.

Once again the medical profession jumped to conclusions and got it wrong

You may be wondering, considering the important functions germanium carries out in your body, why you haven't heard of it before now. This is mainly to do with the bad press germanium received several years ago, regarding reports of toxicity and liver damage following its use.

However, these reports came from people who were irresponsibly given doses that were 20 times the recommended dose for a period of three years without a break – which in effect, caused them to experience serious overdoses.

Any substance when taken in excessive amounts can be dangerous and cause severe health complications – even water can be fatal if this theory is taken to the extreme but, as we know, water is also essential to our health if drunk in moderation.

Fortunately, the original reports have finally been re-evaluated and certain doctors now admit that the scare stories had been based on misinformation that hadn't explored the full story *(Ren Fail 1991, 13(1): 1-4)*.

If taken properly at the correct dose (150mg, one to three times a day) for short periods (up to two months at a time, followed by a break of a month or two – this gives the body enough time to readjust itself), germanium is in fact both safe and extremely effective *(Regul Toxicol Pharmacol 1997, 25(3): 211-219)*.

Germanium has shown no less than 'miraculous' results in fighting cancer

In Japan, germanium has been used to help treat cancer for the past 30 years. The exact mechanism by which it works to tackle cancer has now been uncovered.

Researchers found that germanium reduces the spread of cancer by slowing down the process that causes cancer cells to multiply. At the same time, the researchers observed that germanium didn't interfere with normal, healthy cells, which were left alone to grow and carry out their functions as nature intended *(Chun Hua Yen 2000, 36(4): 263-266)*.

Two years ago a case study confounded many scientists and other members of the medical profession. It involved a patient suffering from a very rare and highly malignant form of lung cancer, called spindle cell carcinoma. Even with radical surgery, combined with radiotherapy and chemotherapy, only a small percentage of patients with this condition live more than a couple of years.

This particular patient had shown no initial response to any of the conventional treatments, and decided to take germanium supplements as a last resort instead. Doctors were astounded to find that even after four years, X-rays showed that the patient was completely free of cancer and that the disease didn't return *(Chest 2000, 117(2): 591-593)*.

Germanium helps protect your body from harmful toxins

Although germanium enhances the action of oxygen in your cells, it also acts as an antioxidant. This means that it is able to reduce the extent of the damage caused by toxic by-products of oxygen metabolism, which takes place in your body. So, in effect it has a double action: both stimulating oxygen use for better health and reducing oxygen's harmful side effects.

Scientists have also found that germanium helps protect the liver's DNA against toxic damage, in addition to increasing the levels of other beneficial antioxidants, such as one called superoxide dismutase *(J Toxicol Environ Health 1999, 58(5): 289-297)*.

Other research findings have demonstrated that used alongside zinc, germanium has an even greater protective effect against free radical damage *(Zhonghuan Yu Fang 1996, 30(4): 221-224)*.

Germanium can even improve the performance of orthodox treatments

Germanium stimulates several components of your immune system. For example, it enhances the activity of macrophages and natural killer cells, both of which are responsible for attacking foreign bacteria and viruses.

It also stimulates the production of gamma interferon, a potent immune molecule (a lymphokine), which is nowadays used by some doctors to fight against severe immune conditions, such as AIDS. Gamma interferon modulates immune reactions particularly against viruses *(Biother 1992, 4(1): 1-8)*.

In studies involving patients suffering from immunological diseases, such as rheumatoid arthritis, lupus and myasthenia (progressive muscle weakness), it was found that germanium acts both as an immune system booster and as an antioxidant.

Conventional treatment of these diseases often involves the drug prednisolone (a steroid hormone). When germanium was given alongside this drug it was found to significantly enhance the actions of prednisolone, making the combined treatment far more powerful and effective against these chronic medical conditions *(Biother 1992, 4(1): 1-8)*.

How to take germanium safely

It's important to take an organic form of germanium to achieve the best results. A good quality form of organic germanium is germanium sesquioxide (the full chemical name which sometimes appears on the box is 'bis-beta-carboxyethyl germanium sesquioxide').

The dose is 150mg one to three times a day, taken between meals. As mentioned above, you shouldn't take this continually. Instead, it's generally recommended that you take germanium for about two months, followed by a break of a month or two should you decide to repeat the process.

• The plant that cancer researchers believe could hail a breakthrough in the fight against the disease

The stem, bark and roots of a rare, succulent, climbing shrub that grows predominantly in India are currently causing a great deal of excitement among cancer researchers.

While its cancer-fighting properties are only just being investigated, *Tinospora cordifolia* – also known as 'guduchi' or heartleaf moonseed – has long been used by Ayurvedic (ancient Indian) practitioners to treat everything from fever and inflammation to diabetes, jaundice and joint pains. It is even sometimes used as an antidote to snake bites and scorpion stings.

Tinospora is what is known as a 'Rasayana' by traditional healers, who credit it with being able to reduce stress, increase vitality and even slow down the ageing process.

It is hardly surprising that tinospora has so many therapeutic properties given its seemingly endless list of beneficial, active ingredients – these include sesquiterpenes, sterols, diterpenes, giloin, gilenin and gilosterol, together with columbin, chasmanthin and palmarin.

Tinospora helps strengthen your body's natural defences

While investigating tinospora's medicinal properties, US scientists from the Miami Children's Hospital found that the plant is able to strengthen the immune system. Their research revealed that it is able to do this by stimulating the action of macrophages – special cells that make up an important part of your body's defence system because of their ability to identify and destroy any infectious bacteria that may be present in your blood.

In addition, the researchers found that the plant reduces the production of a chemical called tumour necrosis factor (TNF), which causes inflammation and your cells to die prematurely *(Int Immunopharmacol. 2006 Dec 5; 6(12): 1815-24)*. This finding helps validate the use of tinospora in Ayurvedic medicine to treat inflammatory disorders like arthritis.

Indian scientists have found that tinospora stimulates other important immune cells such as neutrophils – like macrophages, they also seek out and destroy infectious bugs in your body *(Indian J Exp Biol. 2006 Sep; 44(9): 726-32)*.

Another way the plant works to fortify the immune system is by regulating the activity of cytokines – these proteins play a crucial role in an immune response and have the power to stimulate or inhibit cell activation, proliferation and differentiation. Tinospora increases the production of cytokines when needed and decreases them when they're not, which helps improve overall health and keeps illness at bay *(Altern Med Rev. 2006; 11(2): 128-50)*.

An important breakthrough in the fight against cancer

Tinospora's incredible immune-boosting properties is one of the reasons why it is so effective against cancer. A strong immune system is better able to identify any cancerous cells and eliminate them before they have a chance to grow and spread.

But the plant's anti-cancer benefits don't end there. For example, Indian scientists from the Department of Radiobiology, Kasturba Medical College, have revealed that tinospora extracts contain a chemical called dichloromethane, which is known to poison and kill cancerous cells *(Altern Med. 2006 Jun; 3(2): 267-72)*.

The scientists found that the plant is particularly effective against cancer of the liver. In an animal experiment, they found that the survival rate of mice with liver cancer who received tinospora extracts was improved by a staggering 100 per cent – meaning that the mice with cancer enjoyed the same life expectancy as healthy mice *(Biol Pharm Bull. 2006 Mar; 29(3): 460-6)*.

This finding was backed up by another group of scientists who reported that… "tinospora administration retarded tumour growth and prolonged survival of tumour-bearing mice" *(Immunopharmacol Immunotoxicol. 2005; 27(4): 585-99)*.

In separate research, scientists have found that extracts from the root of the plant contain potent cancer-fighting antioxidants such as catalase, glutathione and superoxide dismutase *(Phytomedicine. 2006 Jan; 13(1-2): 74-84)*.

What to take for best results

As a tincture (i.e. mixed with small amounts of alcohol) the recommended dosage for tinospora is 2-4ml taken twice a day. However, you should be aware that this dosage amount is intended to be used as a guide only, and it is important that you follow the manufacturer's dosage instructions on each individual product, as these can vary.

There are no known contraindications or side effects, although pregnant women and nursing mothers are advised not to take tinospora, as its safety has not been confirmed in these areas.

- **Discover the latest research finding that led one leading scientist to claim is: "The most significant breakthrough in nutrition since the discovery of vitamins"**

In the last couple of decades scientists have begun to uncover hundreds of beneficial compounds in natural foods collectively known as phytonutrients (or phytochemicals). These plant compounds are an emerging area of nutrition that is generating a great deal of excitement amongst scientists.

Although they are not essential for life like traditional nutrients such as protein, vitamins and minerals, they have been shown to play an important role in helping to protect the body against a diverse range of chronic diseases including cancer.

The latest exciting discovery in the field of phytonutrition are substances called salvestrols, which many researchers believe could be one of the most important groups of dietary compounds in the fight against cancer.

Salvestrols are naturally produced in plants in order to protect themselves from attackers such as insects and fungi. It is believed that animals and humans have evolved to make use of these compounds ingested in the diet to help ensure that cells function correctly. In fact, the British scientists that discovered salvestrols have deduced that the protective mechanism of these components was probably developed in mammals around 150 million years ago.

How salvestrols act as a 'Trojan horse' when confronted with cancerous cells

In research published in the *British Naturopathic Journal*, Dan Burke, Emeritus Professor of Pharmaceutical Metabolism, and Gerry Potter, Professor of Medicinal Chemistry who works at De Montfort University in Leicester, explain how salvestrols work *(Salvestrols – natural plant-derived anticancer agents? British Naturopathic Journal Volume 2006; 23:1).*

Their research has revealed that human cells affected by cancer contain an enzyme called CYP1B1. Salvestrols appear to be converted by this enzyme into compounds which can destroy the diseased cells. Because the CYP1B1 enzyme is not present in healthy cells, salvestrols exert no effects there.

"CYP1B1 is a kind of Trojan horse inside the cancer cells," says Professor Burke. "Provide it with salvestrols in the diet and it will unleash a stream of chemical agents that are deadly to the cancer cells."

One of the first salvestrols to be identified was resveratrol – a phytonutrient present in grapes and red wine that is also known for its antioxidant properties *(British Journal of Cancer, 2002; 86: 774-778)*. Other, more powerful salvestrols have now been found in a variety of fruits and vegetables.

For example, they are particularly rich in many red and green coloured health-giving foods such as strawberries, cranberries, raspberries, apples, pears, avocados, broccoli and cabbage. Olives are another excellent source of salvestrols and a number of herbs contain substantial levels including basil, parsley, sage, rosemary, thyme and mint.

Why you shouldn't rely on your diet alone to provide optimum levels of these beneficial plant compounds

With fruit and vegetables being the main dietary source of salvestrols you'd think that people who eat their five a day would be able to obtain all the salvestrols they need for good health. But the latest research findings have revealed that salvestrol levels vary in even the healthiest of diets.

This is because plants make salvestrols for the purpose of pest protection and with the use of modern fungicides and other chemicals, crops do not express salvestrols because they are not exposed to the attacks which cause the plant to produce them in the first place.

Professor Burke says: "Fruit and vegetable plants have evolved over the years to fight off the fungi by generating salvestrol compounds. When we eat the plants we also ingest the salvestrols and derive health benefits.

"But when crops are regularly treated with agrochemical fungicides the plants are rarely exposed to fungus, so they are never stimulated to make salvestrols and the fruit and vegetable harvest lacks these compounds."

According to the researchers, our diets contain probably only 10 per cent of the salvestrol content it did a century ago. Research also indicates that levels of salvestrols are up to 30 times higher in some organic produce, but almost absent in some commercially grown varieties. So opting for organic produce over conventionally produced fruit and vegetables is an effective way of improving salvestrol intake.

Even then there are varying amounts of salvestrols in different varieties of the same fruits and vegetables. This is due to the fact that salvestrols tend to have a bitter taste, so food sources that would normally contain these compounds are being bred to taste sweeter and as a result their salvestrol content is reduced. In addition, cooking may also destroy some of the more fragile salvestrols.

Salvestrol supplements can benefit everything from your skin to your blood pressure

As well as eating organically, another way of boosting levels of salvestrols, which Professor Burke has described as "the most significant breakthrough in nutrition since the discovery of vitamins" is through supplementation.

Fortunately, these cancer-targeting compounds are now available in supplement form derived from organic plant sources. While the main area of salvestrol research has been focused on their anti-cancer potential, people who have been supplementing their diets with these compounds are now reporting other benefits in areas of skin health, blood pressure and anti-fungal activity.

Professor Burke says: "I have received many reports from members of the public who have adopted a high salvestrol regime for a while that they are being helped with various complaints including eczema, psoriasis, high blood pressure, candidiasis and thrush. While we don't know the actual mechanism behind these benefits, we are fairly sure it is not the same mechanism as the anti-cancer effects exerted by salvestrols."

What to take for best results

The recommended dosage for salvestrol is one capsule taken daily with food or as otherwise advised by a healthcare professional. There are no known contraindications when taken at the recommended dosage.

• How to take full advantage of pomegranate's anti-cancer and anti-inflammatory properties

There's an excellent reason for all of the hype that's built up around pomegranates. They've been found to reduce inflammation, fight tumour formation, boost heart health, and protect your vision.

The word is out – and the trend has definitely caught on. On the bright side, that means you're spoiled for choice when it comes to picking out a pomegranate product. But it also means that the door is now wide open for anyone looking to make a quick profit off of this industry darling's new super-fruit status. Before we tell you about a high quality pomegranate supplement, here's the lowdown on this fruit's remarkable anti-cancer properties.

The cancer-fighting phytochemicals you'll only find in pomegranates

Pomegranates are an antioxidant powerhouse, packed with polyphenolic compounds like flavonoids (especially anthocyanins, which give the pulp its rich red colour) and hydrolysable tannins (which can also be found in green tea and red wine). Among the most important polyphenols in pomegranates, though, is a class of tannins called ellagitannins – the compounds responsible for (among other things) the formation of ellagic acid.

Ellagic acid is one of your greatest allies in the fight against cancer. In-vitro studies have demonstrated its ability to inhibit the growth of various types of cancer cells (including breast, colon, and prostate) and to shrink existing tumours by means of apoptosis (programmed cell death) *(J Nutr Biochem. 2004 Nov; 15(11): 672-8).*

But unfortunately, free ellagic acid is of little use in a clinical context, as it demonstrates minimal (if any) antioxidant activity under these conditions. It's virtually unusable to your body in this synthetic form (and may actually result in potentially serious side effects, such as heightened blood pressure).

When bound to glucose in the form of natural ellagitannins, however, its efficacy as a cancer-fighting antioxidant is increased substantially. That's because ellagitannins are extremely water-soluble and bioavailable – and when consumed, your body will synthesize its own ellagic acid as a natural by-product of digestion. This is why fruits that contain these ellagitannins – such as blueberries, strawberries, raspberries... and yes, pomegranates – have assumed a key nutritional role in the prevention and treatment of cancer.

But since every plant has a different phytochemical structure, it's important to note that the most active components of each are bound to differ. In fact, it's actually one particular family of ellagitannins known as punicosides (and specifically punicalagin – both of which are terms derived from the fruit's latin name, *Punica granatum*) that have been pegged as the primary polyphenols at work in pomegranates – not ellagic acid, as once thought *(Eur J Nutr. 2003 Jan; 42(1): 18-28)*.

Researchers now recognise that these punicalagins work synergistically with the ellagic acid they help to form in the human body, thereby delivering the results that we've seen in so many studies *(J Nutr Biochem. 2005 Jun; 16(6): 360-7)*. And it's this total picture that accounts for pomegranate's demonstrated ability to (among other things) fight tumours.

Processing makes (almost) perfect

There's no doubting the health benefits a daily dose of pomegranates can provide. And when it comes down to a choice between eating the fruit and drinking its juice, you might expect that the first of these two options would be most beneficial – after all, fruit is almost always healthier for you than juice alone, thanks to the extra bit of fibre that comes with it.

But this is one of those rare cases when, unless you plan to eat the entire pomegranate (rind and all), you're actually better off going with the juice – that is, assuming that it's commercially prepared.

One study published in the *Journal of Agricultural and Food Chemistry* showed that commercially prepared juice has higher antioxidant activity than home-made juices obtained from the arils (sacks of pulp) alone.

Further analysis revealed that commercial juices contained substantial amounts of punicalagin, while the juice prepared from the arils showed only trace amounts of this ellagitannin. The researchers concluded that additional hydrolysable tannins in the pomegranate's skin are extracted during commercial processing *(J Agric Food Chem. 2000 Oct; 48(10): 4581-9).*

None of this is to say, of course, that there's no benefit in eating pomegranate, or drinking juice that you've prepared for yourself – it simply means that eating the entire fruit is the only way to prevent perfectly good polyphenols from going to waste.

Besides, most of the studies that confirm the healing powers of pomegranate are based around the fruit's juice anyway – so all in all, one cup of pure pomegranate juice a day is probably the most reliable form of this antioxidant that you can get. Nevertheless, there's a major drawback to this mode of delivery: the juice's natural sugar and calorie content.

One eight-ounce glass will set you back a substantial 160 calories and 34g of sugar. And while in the grand scheme of things this may seem like a fair trade, the compromise is far more problematic if you're diabetic. In this case, your best bet is to opt for pomegranate in supplement form instead.

Pomegranate supplements – know what to look for on the label

Make sure you find a supplement made from whole pomegranates, as opposed to an ellagic acid extract – a tip that makes a lot of sense based on what we've already said about synthetic versions of this polyphenol. For this same reason, a supplement containing a complete ellagitannin complex is far more desirable than one containing additional ellagic acid that has already been synthesized in a laboratory – as this could degrade the effectiveness of the pomegranate supplement overall.

All of this also suggests, of course, that you probably shouldn't buy a product that is standardised to a percentage of ellagic acid. While it is indeed an important aspect of pomegranate's antioxidant profile, it's only in the greater context of the fruit's total punicosides (such as in the form of juice, or a whole-fruit extract) that its presence is noteworthy in a supplement *(J Med Food. 2006 Spring; 9(1): 119-22)*. So, look for a product that is standardized to these punicosides instead.

You'll also find a lot of products on the market that include pomegranate as part of a long list of ingredients. But watch out as it's not uncommon for manufacturers to pass off deceptively small amounts of any given ingredient in the guise of their own 'proprietary blend'.

The bottom line: Be wary of any pomegranate formula that doesn't list the exact amount of extract present in each dosage on the label, because you might not be getting much of the good stuff at all. One reputable pomegranate product is Pomegranate Extract Capsules manufactured by LEF.

- ## Rhodiola rosea has a wide range of health benefits and may even protect against cancer

Rhodiola rosea is a perennial plant with yellow or red flowers that grows in cold, mountainous regions of the world. It is held in high regard in Russia, where it is more commonly referred to as 'Golden root', due to the fact that it has been used for centuries to help people cope with the harsh Siberian climate and inhospitable conditions.

It is what herbalists' class as an 'adaptogen' – a herbal remedy that helps promote balance and which is particularly effective at helping to reduce stress levels whilst simultaneously boosting energy and endurance levels.

In fact, rhodiola is fast proving to be one of the most promising adaptogens and is commonly used by Russian athletes to boost their stamina, fight fatigue and help them stay mentally alert and focused. The plant also has many other benefits and has been found to improve cognitive function and memory, promote restful sleep, and speed up the recovery process following an operation or illness.

Studies reveal that rhodiola may help protect against cancer

It is the high concentration of plant chemicals called 'salidrosides' and 'rosavins' in rhodiola, which are thought to be largely responsible for its numerous health-giving properties. Rosavins in particular are known to be extremely effective at fighting several toxins that are found in the environment or are produced by your body in response to stress *(J Chromatogr A. 2005 Dec 9; [Epub ahead of print])*.

Research findings from the Institute of Biological Chemistry, University of Urbino in Italy, have helped shed some light on how rhodiola is effective against outside stressors. The scientists found that the plant is an antioxidant that helps protect red blood cells from environmental toxins, such as heavy metals and free radicals, that are known to damage them *(Eur J Histochem. 2005 Jul-Sep; 49(3): 243-54)*.

Further exciting research conducted at the Department of Plant Morphogenesis, Warsaw University in Poland, suggests that rhodiola may also protect human tissue against cancer.

Not only did the scientists find that the plant helps shield DNA against several toxins implicated in causing cancer, their findings also indicated that the plant may help the body eliminate cancerous cells that are already present *(J Ethnopharmacol. 2006; 103(1): 43-52)*.

What to take for best results

It is important to be aware that there are currently some *Rhodiola rosea* products on the market that are not as strong or effective as claimed on the label. The reason for this is that the plant is very sensitive to changes in temperature, cultivation and collection methods, and is liable to over-drying.

To obtain the maximum benefits to your health therefore, it is important to take a standardised extract of the plant, as this guarantees that the strength of the preparation is constant in every tablet. So make sure you check the product's label for the concentration of the active ingredients: the preparation should contain approximately 3 per cent rosavins and 1 per cent salidroside *(Phytother Res. 2005; 19(9): 740-3)*.

Take 200mg to 600mg of standardised *Rhodiola rosea* root extract per day. It is best to take the tablets before meals and with water.

No harmful side effects or interactions have been reported following its use, but as a precaution it is best not to take rhodiola during pregnancy or while breast-feeding as no studies have been conducted as yet to confirm its safety in these areas.

• Haelan 951 – a revolutionary new type of soya drink that could offer vital protection against cancer

Traditional Chinese Medicine has long recognised the medicinal value of soya beans, and here too in the West they have been widely studied for their ability to prevent certain cancers – especially those of the breast and prostate gland.

Now, an exciting new fermented soya formula, Haelan 951 (which is available as a beverage) appears to offer a high level of protection against cancer and may also be a useful supporting treatment for people who already suffer from the disease.

What makes the formula so exciting is that as well as containing soya, it also contains other powerful natural anti-cancer compounds, which increases its cancer-fighting potential even more.

How does soya help ward off cancer?

Plant chemicals known as isoflavones are thought to play a key role in soya's amazing cancer-preventing qualities. One isoflavone in particular, genistein, has been found to be effective in slowing the progression of prostate cancer.

In a study conducted at the University of California in the US, scientists added genistein to a culture of human prostate cancer cells. It was found to spur the production of a gene called p21, which inhibits the manufacture of a protein that cancer cells need to grow, so causing the cancer cells to die off. Animal studies have confirmed that genistein can reduce the size of prostate cancer tumours *(Health Scout News, June 8, 2001)*.

Isoflavones could prove to be important in preventing against breast cancer too. When 144 women with early breast cancer were matched with healthy controls (same age and area of residence), blood and urine analysis revealed a substantial reduction in breast cancer risk among those who had a high intake of plant isoflavones *(Lancet 1997; 350: 990-4)*.

In another study, pre-menopausal women who ate 60g of soya protein every day for a month showed hormonal and menstrual cycle changes associated with a reduced risk of breast cancer *(Am J Clin Nutr 1994; 60: 333-40)*. The soya isoflavones genistein and daidzein are also antioxidants that help prevent cancer-triggering damage in the body's cells *(Cancer Lett 2001; 172(1): 1-6)*.

Fermented soya products like Haelan 951 have the highest levels of cancer-fighting nutrients

One problem, until the development of the fermentation process, was that these beneficial isoflavones are only present in fairly small amounts in unfermented soya products. For example, a recent Japanese study has found that the level of genistein in fermented soya products is far higher than in unfermented soya beans, soya milk or tofu *(J Agric Food Chem 2001 Jun; 49(6): 2839-43).*

The fermentation process involves turning a food into a healthier product by adding ingredients that have known health benefits. The fermentation process used to produce traditional Japanese soya foods such as miso, tempeh and natto enormously increases the availability of isoflavones. It is thought to do this by converting precursor chemicals called genistin and daidzin to their active anti-cancer isoflavone forms, genistein and daidzein *(Carcinogenesis 1995; 16(3): 471-6).*

However, getting hold of fermented soya foods and making them a regular part of a Western diet can be difficult. That's what makes Haelan 951 such a breakthrough product, as it contains all the benefits of fermented soya foods in a convenient drink. It is a concentrated nutritional supplement that, as well as containing high levels of genistein and daidzein, is rich in many other beneficial nutrients – up to 20 of which may also have cancer-fighting properties, such as branched-chain fatty acids, phytates, phytosterols, saponins and protease inhibitors.

Prostate tumour growth inhibited by up to 50%

Animal studies examining the anti-cancer potential of the fermented soya phytochemicals (natural plant chemicals) in Haelan 951, were carried out by US scientists at the University of Southern California.

The researchers discovered that one of the active anti-cancer agents in the formula, a group of branched-chain fatty acids called small biosynthetic anti-cancer agents (SBA) reduced prostate cancer cell size and cell growth, as well as reducing the formation of blood vessels in prostate tumours that are needed to support its growth.

The study also investigated the effects of SBA on laboratory cultures of human prostate cancer cells. They found that tumour formation was inhibited by 50 per cent, indicating a strong anti-tumour activity *(Cancer Research, 2000; 60: 505-509).*

There are at least five other main anti-cancer agents in Haelan951. Firstly, several isoflavones have strong inhibiting effects in hormone-related malignancies such as prostate, ovarian, cervical and breast cancers. Secondly, compounds known as phytates bind iron in the intestines to prevent it from generating free radicals, which have been shown to result in malignancies.

Thirdly, phytosterols are known to neutralise the breakdown products of cholesterol and so reduce the development of certain types of cancers. Fourthly, saponins stop the cellular mutations that could lead to malignancy. Lastly, protease inhibitors are able to prevent the activation of mutant cancer-causing genes called oncogenes *(Well Being Journal 2002; 11(6))*.

How Haelan 951 may prove effective against recurrent cases of prostate cancer

US cancer specialists at the Prostate Cancer Research and Education Foundation in California carried out a small trial in 1998 with 12 patients who all had a history of recurrent prostate cancer and rising levels of prostate specific antigen (PSA) – an indicator of the severity of the disease. All of the patients were given a fermented soya drink, in this case Haelan 851 (an earlier version of Haelan 951). The researchers found that half of the patients in the study responded to the treatment with a drop in their PSA levels.

Individual case studies also support the effectiveness of Haelan 951. One 58-year-old man was first diagnosed with a prostate tumour following a biopsy three years ago. His doctor recommended either surgery to remove his prostate gland, or radiotherapy. The patient refused both options and instead started taking Haelan 951, two weeks after receiving the diagnosis. His PSA levels have remained stable for three years and, at his last check-up, his prostate gland appeared perfectly normal on rectal examination and ultrasound scan *(Well Being Journal 2002; 11(6))*.

What to use for best results

The recommended preventative dosage for Haelan 951 is one to two tablespoons a day. Higher dosage amounts would be required for treatment purposes and would need to be determined by a practitioner familiar with the product.

- **Boost your immune system with "the most powerful immune complex... ever tested!"**

It has long been known that the key to good health is a strong and fully-functioning immune system. That's why scientists at the cutting edge of naturopathic medicine are constantly searching for safe and effective natural immune-boosters to maximise your body's ability to fight disease.

Research to date shows that BioBran MGN-3® can help people with serious conditions, such as cancer, AIDS, diabetes, hepatitis B and C, and chronic fatigue syndrome *(Williams, David G, A New Chapter in Healing, Alternatives Vol. 7 No. 15, p.117, September 1998)*.

Dr Mamdooh Ghoneum, a professor at the Department of Immunology at Drew University of Medicine and Science in the US, has spent the last 20 years researching immune system boosters. He describes BioBran as: "The most powerful immune complex I have ever tested!"

So impressed was he with the results that Dr Ghoneum has now devoted his entire research efforts to treatments with this compound. Developed and manufactured in Japan, BioBran is made from the breakdown or pre-digestion of rice bran with enzymes from the health-giving shiitake mushroom – it is well absorbed by the body with no reported side effects.

Studies show BioBran helps boost cancer-fighting cells by up to 300%!

Your immune system is made up of various white blood cells (WBCs) – including natural killer (NK) cells, T-cells and B-cells. The job of the NK cells and T-cells is to destroy potentially hazardous microbes that penetrate your body's defences, as well as infected or abnormal (cancer) cells. The role of B-cells is to produce antibodies to attack invading micro-organisms or neutralise toxic substances.

BioBran works by stimulating the overall activity of your immune system, especially your NK cells. In fact, BioBran has been clinically proven to increase NK cell activity by as much as 300 per cent *(International Journal of Immunotherapy 1998; XIV(2): 89-99)*.

NK cells are your body's first line of defence against cancer and viral infection and research shows that individuals with low NK cell activity are more likely to develop cancer or virally-related diseases *(Clinical Immunotherapeutics 1994; 1(1): 56-66)*. BioBran also boosts the activity of the T-cells and B-cells by up to 200 per cent *(Ghoneum, M. Effect of MGN-3 on Human Natural Killer Cell Activity and Interferon-γ Synthesis in Vitro, FASEB 1996; 10(6): 26-32)*.

Because of its immune-boosting powers, BioBran is the perfect supplement to conventional cancer therapies (chemotherapy and radiotherapy). Doctors have found that patients with leukaemia and multiple myeloma (plasma cell cancer) show the greatest response to BioBran. However, ovarian, prostate and breast cancer sufferers have also done well on this supplement.

BioBran can activate your body's defences in just under 2 weeks

In one trial undertaken by Dr Ghoneum and Dr J Brown, at the Drew University of Medicine and Science, 32 patients who had previously completed conventional cancer therapy for different types of advanced cancers each received a course of BioBran.

Before the trial, the baseline NK cell activity was found to be low in all participants (10.8 per cent – 49 per cent). After only two weeks on BioBran there was a significant increase in NK cell activity. This ranged from 145 per cent to 332 per cent in breast cancer patients, 174 per cent to 385 per cent in prostate cancer patients and 100 per cent to 537 per cent in multiple myeloma patients. NK cell activity was maintained for five years with continued use of BioBran *(Ghoneum M, Manantalla G. NK Immunomodulatory Function in 27 Patients by MGN-3, a Modified Arabinoxylan from Rice Bran. Abstract, 87th Meeting of the American Association for Cancer Research, April 1996, Washington DC).*

A second study by Dr Ghoneum monitored five women with breast cancer. After being treated with BioBran, four out of the five women have experienced disease remission *(Ghoneum M. Immunomodulatory and Anticancer Properties of MGN-3, a Modified Xylose from Rice Bran, in Five Patients with Breast Cancer. Abstract, American Association for Cancer Research Special Conference; The Interface Between Basic and Applied Research, Nov 1995, Baltimore, MD).* (The researchers were unable to report on how the fifth patient got on as they lost contact with her).

"Long-term stabilisation or remission of disease in the large majority of cases"

These studies and others undertaken by Dr Ghoneum (in animals and humans) show that BioBran is efficient in activating NK cells. A single NK cell can destroy up to 27 cancer cells before it dies.

Dr Ghoneum reports that "the documented increase in NK cell activity in cancer patients taking BioBran has been correlated to dramatic reductions in corresponding tumour markers and other pathology indicators, and, most importantly, to long-term stabilisation or remission of disease in the large majority of cases."

However, Dr Ghoneum is adamant that BioBran is no substitute for 'debulking therapies' (chemotherapy, radiation or surgery) especially in cases of advanced malignancies.

"I recommend that cancer patients with solid tumours begin BioBran immunotherapy concurrent with, or immediately following debulking therapies," he says. "This gives BioBran its best chance to get rid of those cancer cells that escaped the debulking therapy, and keep them from ever coming back."

What to take for best results

The recommended dose for BioBran MGN-3® varies from 500mg to 3,000mg a day with food. For health maintenance 500mg a day is sufficient. Those advised by their medical practitioner to take a higher dosage may use 3,000mg a day for eight weeks (1,000mg after each meal) and then 1,000mg a day thereafter.

- **Discover how a weed is offering hope to countless cancer sufferers**

Bindweed, or *Convolvulus arvensis*, is a farmer's nightmare, strangling crops by twining itself around them – and because of this, it has earned itself the nickname 'the cancer of weeds'. Yet, ironically, many scientists now believe that substances isolated from this amazing botanical powerhouse offer real hope for cancer sufferers.

Biochemicals extracted from bindweed have been shown to shut down the blood supply to cancerous tumours, effectively cutting off nutrients and oxygen needed by the malignant cells.

Remarkably, the biochemicals it contains have been shown to be a hundred times more effective at starving the tumours than shark cartilage, another natural supplement that has shown potential in the treatment of cancer (*Riordan NH, Meng X and Riordan HD, Research paper presented at Comprehensive Cancer Care 2000, Arlington, Virginia, June 2000*).

Bindweed extract has also been found to be beneficial in stimulating the immune system to produce more white blood cells, which have the power to destroy cancer cells. And now, after a breakthrough in the extraction process, bindweed extract has become available in supplement form in the UK.

Studies began after claims about bindweed's cancer-fighting powers

Interest in bindweed was triggered in 1994 when a cancer patient turned up at the offices of scientist Neil Riordan, at the Center for the Improvement of Human Functioning in Wichita, Kansas.

In 1987, the woman had been diagnosed with ovarian cancer and given just a year to live. Conventional treatment offered her little hope so she had sought help from alternative practitioners instead, including an Indian shaman (medicine man) in Oklahoma where she lived. The shaman gave her a traditional Indian remedy, known as tincture of bindweed.

Seven years on from that grim diagnosis, the woman told Neil Riordan that she remained in good health and that her cancer, astonishingly, was reportedly under control. Now she wanted to share her remarkable story with others, so that they too might benefit from bindweed's extraordinary powers.

Active ingredient found to prevent the spread of tumours by up to 73%

Struck by the woman's remarkable testimony, Neil Riordan and his research team started investigating the mechanism by which bindweed might combat cancer.

Some tumours rely on a dense network of blood vessels – a development known as angiogenesis – to fuel their growth and spread. The scientists soon discovered that bindweed stopped new blood vessels from growing to and from the tumour site.

In laboratory tests, Riordan's team identified the active ingredients as proteoglycans. They were found to prevent angiogenesis by up to 73 per cent. The researchers also found that the proteoglycan mixture stimulated the immune system to produce more white blood cells, or lymphocytes, which are able to devour cancer cells. Tests showed a significant increase in lymphocyte activity of between 35 per cent and 46 per cent *(Riordan NH, Meng X and Riordan HD, Research paper presented at Comprehensive Cancer Care 2000, Arlington, Virginia, June 2000).*

Bindweed extract was then examined in a number of clinical trials involving cancer patients – and there are some remarkable testimonies to its power.

Bindweed extract has given some cancer patients a second chance

One woman, a 62-year-old nurse with inoperable pancreatic cancer who had been given just three months to live, was delighted to be told that her tumour had shrunk dramatically after she started taking bindweed extract. "A walking miracle" is how one doctor described her *(Schwontkowski D, A Weed with a Purpose: Bindweed and Cancer, www.stopcancer.com/drdonna.htm).*

Another 57-year-old woman, with breast cancer that had metastasised (spread) from its original site to her lung, brain and bones, had been having chemotherapy for four months without showing any improvement. Just two months after starting to take bindweed extract, her brain lesions had disappeared and the lung metastases had reduced by 50 per cent *(Focus [Allergy Research Group Newsletter], March 2001).*

Another 'terminal' breast cancer patient, with metastases in the liver and bones, saw her tumours shrink by almost half, during the first six weeks of taking bindweed extract *(Focus [Allergy Research Group*

Newsletter], March 2001).

The safety and efficacy of bindweed extract has earned the praise of many practitioners

The doctors and nutritional therapists who have pioneered its use are unanimous in their praise for bindweed extract. Mary Shackelton ND, of Boulder, Colorado, says: "Bindweed proteoglycan mixture seems to be responsible for a lot of positive changes in my patients' cancer treatment. My patients also report that they feel better and experience a reduction of symptoms after taking bindweed."

Dr Julian Kenyon MD, MB, ChB, Medical Director of the Dove Clinic for Integrative Medicine in Hampshire, feels that bindweed extract has "a very exciting future" in alternative medical practice. "We have observational clinical evidence so far that it is an effective angiogenesis inhibitor. We also find that it is much better tolerated than shark cartilage."

Bindweed extract has undergone seven years of laboratory tests, animal toxicity trials and clinical observations. Although bindweed, before the extraction process, contains alkaloids that can be poisonous, a method has been developed for commercially extracting just the proteoglycan mixture, which has been shown to be entirely non-toxic.

In animal tests, no adverse effects were seen at the equivalent of 1,400g human dose – the normal therapeutic dose is 0.5 to 1.5g a day. What is more, bindweed extract is often effective where conventional therapies have failed, and it has none of the side effects of chemotherapy and radiotherapy, such as nausea, hair loss and immune suppression.

It is most effective when used as part of a natural cancer care programme and combined with strong immune system stimulants, such as vitamin C. It is important to note that any such treatment programme should be supervised by a doctor or nutritional therapist, and you should not stop taking any prescribed drugs without consulting with your doctor first.

• How a little-known ingredient found in fruit and vegetables can reduce your risk of cancer

The health-giving benefits to be had from following a diet rich in fruit and vegetables, are endlessly reported on in the health pages of newspapers and magazines. Yet what the media has failed to pick up on is an astonishing new discovery that provides an even greater reason to take advantage of this readily available source of good health and longevity.

Scientists have identified an amazing new compound in fresh produce called glucaric acid, which has been shown to exert a powerful anti-cancer effect.

Together with the abundance of antioxidant vitamins, minerals and phytochemicals we know to be present in fresh fruit and vegetables, it makes a stunning health-giving combination.

Apples, apricots, cherries and grapefruit are the richest sources of glucaric acid. Brussels sprouts, broccoli, cabbage, alfalfa sprouts and lettuce, also contain significant levels. In addition, glucaric acid is produced in our bodies in small amounts. However, some researchers believe that taking extra in supplement form – as calcium D-glucarate – can be extremely beneficial.

These health-giving benefits were discovered by researchers at the world-renowned M.D. Anderson Cancer Center in Houston, Texas in the US. They found that supplementation with calcium D-glucarate appears to enhance the detoxification process of harmful chemicals and excess steroid hormones, such as oestrogen – successfully increasing their elimination from your body.

Calcium D-glucarate helps rid your body of cancer-causing substances

Calcium D-glucarate is of particular importance to those who may have a genetic susceptibility to tumour development, or those who expose themselves to cancer-forming substances such as tobacco. (Besides hereditary factors, cancer risk has been associated with a number of lifestyle factors including smoking, excess exposure to sunlight, exposure to environmental chemicals such as pesticides, and poor dietary habits.)

One of the key ways in which your body gets rid of toxic chemicals and excess hormones is by combining them with glucuronic acid in your liver, and then excreting in the bile.

However, this process can be compromised by an enzyme called beta-glucuronidase, which is produced by certain bacteria that reside in your gut. This enzyme breaks the bond between the toxic compound and glucuronic acid – this releasing action means that these toxic chemicals can then be easily reabsorbed into your body, instead of being excreted.

Elevated beta-glucuronidase activity is thought to increase the risk of various cancers – particularly hormone-dependent cancers, like those of the breast and prostate *(Cancer Detect Prev 1997; 21: 178-90 [review]; www.gnc.com)*.

By inhibiting the activity of beta-glucuronidase, calcium D-glucarate helps your body to eliminate various toxic chemicals and hormones, which might otherwise contribute to cancer development.

Calcium D-glucarate can lower the risk of certain cancers by up to 60%

Dr Thomas Slaga, President of the Center for Cancer Causation and Prevention at AMC Cancer Research Center in Denver, in the

US, states: "In individuals at risk for cancer, glucaric acid levels are low and it tends to be excreted quickly from the body. In such individuals, beta-glucuronidase activity is high and there is less excretion of carcinogens and toxins.

"If an individual were to have higher levels of glucaric acid, he or she may be able to slow down the work of the 'bad enzyme' beta-glucuronidase, and rid his or her body of dangerous toxins and carcinogens."

Although more research is needed, laboratory tests carried out so far have shown that calcium D-glucarate can prevent the development of experimentally-induced cancers *(Carcinogenesis 1986; 7: 1463-6; Cancer Lett 1990; 49: 51-7; Cancer Lett 1986; 33(1): 25-32; J Toxicol Environ Health 1988; 23: 15-27)*. Calcium D-glucarate has been shown to decrease lung, skin, liver, breast and colon cancers by 60 per cent or more.

In addition, it has been found to have an inhibitory effect on cancers of the bladder and prostate. In one study, a 50 per cent reduction in beta-glucoronidase activity was associated with a 23 per cent decrease in circulating oestradiol (the most potent form of oestrogen which has been associated with making breast cancer cells multiply) *(Carcinogenesis, 1996; 7(9) 1463-1466)*.

What to take for best results

The suggested dose for calcium D-glucarate is between 200mg and 500mg twice a day. However, higher levels are recommended for individuals with existing cancer. If you have been diagnosed with cancer you should see your healthcare practitioner before starting a supplement regime.

Contraindications: No side effects have been reported following the use of calcium D-glucarate. However, because it encourages the elimination of hormones and toxins it may also increase the elimination of some drugs, thereby reducing their effectiveness. Individuals who are on prescription drugs and wish to take calcium D-glucarate should therefore consult their GP or specialist before use.

• Ashwagandha: Exciting new research findings reveal how the herb can help fight cancer

Scientists are discovering what Ayurvedic (ancient Indian) medical practitioners have known for centuries – that ashwagandha (traditionally known as Indian ginseng), can successfully help combat a diverse range of ailments.

The traditional uses of the herb are as a tonic and invigorator. It is believed to prolong longevity, boost mental and physical stamina, and improve sexual function (which is how it earned the nickname 'herbal viagra').

It has also been used to alleviate stress and anxiety, because it has a calming effect and lowers levels of the hormone cortisol – which is produced in high amounts during stressful situations. Applied directly to the skin the herb can also provide much-needed relief from eczema, psoriasis, wounds and skin ulcers.

The recent studies are particularly exciting as they have uncovered new health benefits attached to ashwagandha – one of the most promising of which is its ability to fight cancer – as well as backing up many of its traditional uses.

Ashwagandha strengthens your immune system and protects against harmful toxins

Your immune system is made up of a complex structure of proteins, cells and chemicals, which work together in harmony to fight bacteria, viruses, cancer and other damage to your tissues.

In trials, extracts from the ashwagandha root were found to boost the functioning of the immune system, making it even more effective and active. This is due, in part, to the root extract's ability to increase the number of white blood cells in your body, which fight invading bacteria and viruses.

The extract also improves the action of platelets which are essential constituents of your blood that promote healthy blood clotting. The glycowithanolide chemicals found in the ashwagandha root, in particular those called withanolides I and II, can significantly lessen any damage caused to your immune system by toxic chemicals, by binding to toxins and eliminating them *(J Ethnopharmacol 1999, 67(1): 27-35).*

On the subject of immunity, scientists from the Department of Biosciences, Vellore Institute of Technology, Deemed University in India, recently found that the herb is able to both regulate the immune system and reduce the risk of inflammation. This latter benefit is particularly important as inflammation is now implicated in a number of serious conditions, including cancer.

Targets cancer cells and encourages their destruction

Research shows that ashwagandha root extract may be able to detect cancerous cells in the body and prevent them from spreading. The extract also performs another important function in that it appears to be able to cut off the blood supply to cancerous cells, thereby causing them to die *(J Ethnopharmacol. 2006 May 24; 105(3): 336-41).*

Further research has revealed that the herb may help cancer sufferers in another way. When patients are undergoing treatment with conventional anti-cancer drugs, chemotherapy or radiotherapy it puts the body under enormous stress.

The fact that ashwagandha has been found to strengthen the immune system means that cancer patients might be better able to withstand the harsh effects associated with these treatments *(Chem Biol Interact. 2006; 159(3): 180-5).*

Ashwagandha can counteract the damage caused by chemotherapy. Patients undergoing chemotherapy for cancer put their body under considerable stress. And scientists are constantly searching for treatments which can help reduce this. Ashwagandha was tested on cells exposed to chemotherapy and radiotherapy, and was shown to be effective in protecting these cells against further damage *(Ind J Exp Biol 1996, 34(10) 927-932)*.

This also has far-reaching implications for helping to protect the tissues of healthy people who are exposed to ordinary toxins and environmental pollutants.

What to take for best results

The recommended dosage for ashwagandha is one 250mg to 300mg capsule taken two or three times a day, preferably with meals. Ashwagandha should not be taken alongside sedatives, alcohol or other stimulants. In addition, pregnant women should not take the herb.

• A new supplement heralds good news for cancer and diabetes sufferers

Scientists have known for some time now that a naturally occurring substance, found in your body's cells and also present in vegetable fibre, is an effective anti-cancer agent. Now, there is mounting evidence to suggest that this active compound could also play a vital role in the prevention and management of Type 2 diabetes.

Inositol hexaphosphate (IP6), also known as phytic acid, is a component of fibre found in whole grains and legumes (peas and beans). However, the quantities of IP6 derived from these dietary sources are too small to provide any real therapeutic value.

Now this problem has finally been overcome following the development of IP6 in supplement form. Taken in this way, more of it can be efficiently absorbed and utilised by your body.

Following a review of numerous study results, US scientists have concluded that IP6 – and its related substance IP3 (formed when IP6 enters your body) – could be the key to regulating healthy insulin production *(American Journal of Physiology Endocrinology and Metabolism, 283, p E1113-E1122)*. Their findings open exciting doors to the future management of diabetes and herald a brighter future for those with a family history of the disease who are trying to prevent its onset in later life.

How cancer research led to this exciting discovery

Naturopath Marcus Webb, who also works as a chartered biologist and technical director at Hadley Wood Healthcare, the company behind the development of IP6, says that the excitement about IP6 and diabetes has come about almost as a "side effect" of the extensive research into IP6 and cancer.

In fact, over the past 15 years, studies on IP6 have mainly focused on its role as an antioxidant and anti-cancer agent. A leader in this field has been Dr Abul Shamsuddin, Professor of Medicine at the University of Maryland School of Medicine, in Baltimore in the US. He and fellow researchers have published a number of key papers on the benefits of IP6 in fighting cancer.

One of the reasons why it is thought to be so effective in this area is due to the fact that it is a powerful antioxidant – meaning that it helps render free radicals harmless, which can otherwise increase the risk of the disease developing.

According to scientists IP6 may also help to inhibit the spread of established cancer, as it has been shown to slow down the rate of abnormal cell division *(International Journal of Food Science and Technology, Vol 37, p 769-782; I Vucenik, AM Shamsuddin. Inhibition of growth and induction of differentiation by IP6. June 2002. European Cancer Research Symposium, Granada, Spain).*

It also boosts immunity by increasing the activity of natural killer cells, which help fight off viruses, bacteria and cancerous cells. Not only that but it may also have the added benefit of preventing the formation of kidney stones *(Laboratory of Renal Lithiasis Research, Faculty of Science, University of Balearic Islands, Palma de Mallorca, Spain, Life Sciences, 16 August 2002, p 1535-1546)*.

Marcus Webb says that in the course of patients taking IP6 for the above medical complaints, researchers noticed that many of them were not only experiencing health-related benefits in these specific areas, but tests were also revealing healthier blood sugar levels.

According to Marcus, IP6 probably helps to benefit health in so many different ways because it appears to play a key role in cell-to-cell communication. He says, "The anecdotal evidence is supported by a good grounding in the theory of how it should work"…"And the more you look into the cellular basis of disease, the more you see that communication between cells is at the roots of it."

"Since I've been taking it, I feel better and I feel fitter… and my blood sugar level has come down"

When IP6 enters the body it divides to produce two molecules of IP3; it is IP3 that plays a major role in the communication between cells. In this new IP6 supplement, IP6 is combined in a four-to-one ratio with inositol (a member of the B-vitamin group), which helps IP6 to create IP3 more efficiently.

IP6 and IP3 help regulate blood sugar levels by encouraging the efficient functioning of beta cells in your pancreas. Scientists know that these cells are sensitive to glucose and are responsible for the process that leads to insulin (which helps regulate glucose) being released. If these cells are not working properly then Type 2 diabetes can occur.

What to take for best results

The recommended dosage is two capsules of IP6 capsules twice a day. In powder form, the suggested dose is one scoop twice a day (see label for further details). There have not been any reports of side effects linked to taking IP6 supplements, but as always check with your doctor if you are currently on medication.

• How to safeguard your health from a diverse range of diseases... including cancer

If you're searching for a safe and effective natural remedy that can improve your overall health as well as offer protection against numerous ailments, then look no further. *Taraxacum officinale*, more commonly known as dandelion extract, is proving to be an excellent all-round remedy.

Taraxacum has been studied extensively during the past few years and has been found to possess a wide range of beneficial actions. Traditionally the roots of the plant have been used against jaundice and gallbladder problems, whereas the leaves are used specifically to reduce fluid retention.

It's little wonder that it is effective against so many conditions when you consider the wealth of ingredients it contains, including flavonoids, vitamins A, C and D, resin, mucilage, magnesium, iron, potassium, inulin and polysaccharides *(J. Phytochemistry 1996; 42: 121-127; Zhongguo Zhong Yao 1999; 24(4): 225-226 Hu).*

They have a synergistic effect and account for taraxacum's multiple health benefits, such as helping to prevent serious conditions like cancer, heart disease and stroke. Its ability to regulate blood sugar levels also makes it beneficial for diabetics.

"Potential as a therapeutic agent in human leukaemia"

Canadian researchers from the Faculty of Agricultural Sciences, at the University of British Columbia, have been studying the antioxidant actions of taraxacum.

They reported, just a few weeks ago, that the extract exerts a potent antioxidant effect. It was found to be particularly beneficial in protecting against DNA damage caused by free radicals. It also reduces free-radical damage to the fat components of cells that, left unchecked, can eventually lead to cell death which accelerates the ageing process and increases the risk of cancer *(I Agric Food Chem 2003; 51(1): 301-310).*

Further exciting research findings have revealed that specific plant chemicals – taraxacin, taraxacerin and taraxinic acid – found in taraxacum, may help in the fight against leukaemia *(Fitotherapia 2000; 71(3): 269-273).*

Korean scientists from the College of Pharmacy, Kyung Hee University in Seoul have reported that taraxinic acid, in particular, is extremely active in destroying cancerous cells in patients suffering from leukaemia. Dr Choi, the principal investigator concluded that: "taraxinic acid may have a potential as a therapeutic agent in human leukaemia" *(Biol Pharm Bull 2002; 25(11): 1446-1450).*

... Its list of health-related benefits just keeps on growing

New research is unveiling several hitherto unknown benefits linked to taraxacum. For example, researchers from the Department of Biological Sciences, University of Ulsan in Korea, have detected a protein molecule in it that acts as an anti-coagulant *(Biosci Biotechnol Biochem 2002; 66(9): 1859-1864).*

The protein stops blood from clotting prematurely and offers promising potential as a preventative against blood clots, which increase the risk of stroke, heart attacks and thrombosis. This clot-busting protein is so new that it hasn't even been given a scientific name yet.

In addition, it's been revealed that taraxacum can block inflammatory chemicals, including interleukin-6 and tumour necrosis factor-alpha (TNF-a), that are implicated in contributing to cancer, arthritis and brain damage *(Immunopharmacol Immunotoxicol 2000; 22(3): 519-530).*

What to take for best results

The recommended dose is 540mg of taraxacum taken one to three times a day. There are no reports of side effects or toxicity. However, you should be aware that people who are allergic to pollen are at risk of suffering an allergic reaction to taraxacum extract.

- ## This incredible Chinese mushroom could slash your risk of cancer

Red reishi *(Ganoderma lucidum)* has long been considered the number one herb in traditional Chinese medicine and is known as the 'mushroom of immortality'. Once reserved solely for the use of emperors, who believed it would grant them eternal youth and good health, it has only recently come to the attention of Western medicine.

After centuries of anecdotal evidence and hundreds of research papers, placebo-controlled clinical trials have now proved reishi's amazing ability to boost the immune system and even fight certain cancers. Other studies also suggest its potential benefits in health problems as diverse as heart disease, diabetes, prostate enlargement and chronic fatigue.

Red reishi is generally considered to be the most potent variety of the reishi mushroom. Now one of the highest quality supplements on the market, Mikei Red Reishi Essence, is available in the UK. Red reishi's effectiveness largely depends on the conditions in which it is cultivated.

The mushrooms for Mikei Red Reishi Essence are grown on carefully selected Japanese aged oak logs, producing one of the most superior red reishi extracts available. More than 200 different substances have been isolated from red reishi, among which polysaccharides and triterpenoids have been identified as the main groups of active components.

Studies indicate that the various polysaccharides are responsible for strengthening and modulating the immune system whereas triterpenoids (of which more than 119 have already been found in red reishi) have direct anti-tumour and anti-inflammatory effects *(Planta Med 2009, 25 Aug [Epub ahead of print])*. Red reishi's other ingredients may also work synergistically to contribute to its disease-fighting effects.

Red reishi powers up the immune system and stops cancer cells in their tracks

Dozens of scientific studies have indicated red reishi's incredible ability to boost general health by supporting the body's immune system. Newly published research from the Academy of Chinese Medical Sciences in Beijing has demonstrated that red reishi extract actually stimulates the creation of specific immune cells (called enteric mucosal lymphocytes and peripheral blood mononuclear cells), as well as increasing the amounts of tumour-fighting substances these cells produce *(Chem Biodivers 2007; 4(2): 224-231)*.

The evidence that reishi can strengthen the immune system is hard to argue against and the Cancer Research Campaign was so intrigued by it that they commissioned a paper looking at oriental mushrooms' ability to help cancer patients, which concluded that "purified bioactive compounds derived from medicinal mushrooms are a potentially important new source of anti-cancer agents" *(Perspectives in Biology and Medicine 2006; 49(2): 159-170)*.

Recent laboratory and animal studies have shown that red reishi extract ends leukaemia cells' growth and proliferation (*Evid Based Complement Alternat Med 2009, 20 Aug [Epub ahead of print]*). In addition to reducing tumour size, it also appears to prevent the metastasis (spreading throughout the body) of liver cancer cells *(J Agric Food Chem 2009; 57(11): 5049-5057)*. In a clinical trial involving 47 patients with advanced colorectal cancer, treatment with red reishi extract for 12 weeks was found to improve markers of immune activity, including numbers of 'natural killer' cells and levels of the natural anti-cancer chemical interferon-gamma *(Int Immunopharmacol 2006; 6(3): 499-508)*.

Red reishi also has a reputation for maintaining a healthy heart and circulation, and research shows it reduces both blood pressure and the levels of fats in the blood *(J Nutr Sci Vitaminol (Tokyo) 1988; 34(4): 433-438)*. Animal studies carried out in Taiwan have revealed that red reishi's antioxidant properties can protect the heart from free radical damage *(Phytother Res 2004; 18(12): 1024-1026)*. What's more, recent work by Russian scientists suggests that red reishi could prevent damage to heart tissue during a heart attack *(Patol Fiziol Eksp Ter 2008; 1: 22-25)*.

Red reishi reduces blood sugar levels

New research from the University of Hong Kong has shown that red reishi could be valuable in the management of diabetes and metabolic syndrome. In mice at least, red reishi switches off a gene responsible for the production of glucose in the liver and in doing so, reduces blood sugar levels *(Phytomedicine 2009; 16(5): 426-436)*.

Interestingly, this is exactly the same mechanism by which the diabetes drug metformin works. A separate study with rats has found that red reishi extract protects the insulin-producing cells in the pancreas from experimentally-induced damage by alloxan, a chemical that selectively destroys these cells *(Life Sci 2003; 73(18): 2307-2319)*.

What to take for best results

Mikei Red Reishi Essence comes in packs of 30 capsules, each containing 250mg of concentrated red reishi essence powder. The recommended dosage is one capsule a day. Women who are pregnant or breastfeeding are advised to consult their doctor before taking Mikei Red Reishi Essence.

- ### Another mushroom that is proving its worth in the fight against cancer is Coriolus versicolor

Coriolus versicolor is an extremely popular cancer treatment in China and Japan, used by both orthodox and alternative practitioners alike. In fact, in 1987, *Coriolus versicolor* extract accounted for more than a quarter of all expenditure on anti-cancer drugs in Japan (*Medicinal Mushrooms: An exploration of Tradition, Healing and Culture by Christopher Hobbs*).

A dietary supplement based on this remarkable mushroom is now available in the UK. At long last, you too can benefit from the potent antioxidant, anti-microbial, antiviral and anti-tumour properties of *Coriolus versicolor*.

Studies into Coriolus versicolor began after reports of its remarkable anti-cancer benefits

Coriolus versicolor, commonly found growing in dead trees in woodlands throughout Europe, North America and Asia, has fan-shaped fruiting bodies which grow in overlapping clusters, said to resemble turkey plumage.

Traditionally, these mushrooms were used to make a sweet-tasting tea. Scientific interest in their medicinal use, however, was triggered more than 30 years ago, after a chemical engineer in Japan decided to investigate the apparent anti-cancer properties of the mushroom.

He had observed that the spread of his neighbour's life-threatening cancer was halted after taking extracts of *Coriolus versicolor*. This culminated in a report claiming that a type of Japanese tea – Saru-no-koshikake, which contains *Coriolus versicolor* – was beneficial for stomach cancer patients.

Mushroom's active ingredient strengthens your immune system to ward off harmful viruses

Numerous studies followed – more than 400 to date – and extracts from *Coriolus versicolor* were shown to be powerful immune system boosters. The therapeutic properties were subsequently linked to a biochemical, christened polysaccharide K (PSK) or krestin, which was extracted from the mushroom's thread-like extensions known as mycelium.

A polysaccharide is a large, complex branched structure made up of smaller sugar molecules. In most mushrooms, including *Coriolus versicolor*, the polysaccharide is bound to a protein.

PSK appears to work by directly stimulating the immune system into producing more natural killer cells, potent white blood cells that protect the body against bacteria, viruses, and a host of damaging environmental toxins.

With regard to its anti-tumour activity, PSK appears to act directly on tumour cells as well as boosting cellular immunity. Animal studies show that it limits the growth of skin, breast, colon and lung cancers *(Tsukagoshi,S. et al. 1984. Krestin (PSK). Cancer Treatment Reviews 11: 131 155)*. It also appears to halt the spread of cancer cells *(Ebina, T.1987b. Antitumour effect of PSK.(2) Effector Mechanism of antimetastatic effect in the 'double grafted tumor system'. Gon to Kagaku Ryobo 14: 1847-1853. From CA 107: 10896lf)*.

New research suggests Coriolus versicolor has potent cancer-fighting abilities

Coriolus versicolor is being investigated for its ability to treat cervical dysplasia – cell abnormalities in the cervix that may develop into cancerous cells. Around 90 per cent of all cervical cancers are linked to infection with the Human Papillomavirus (HPV). This is a commonly occurring virus and about 80 per cent of women are infected with it within four years of becoming sexually active.

Dr Monro believes that the antiviral properties of PSK, together with its ability to boost natural killer cell production, offers hope of a safe, non-surgical treatment option.

PSK has been used orally and intravenously in cancer management since 1970 by orthodox and alternative practitioners, most commonly for cancers of the stomach, oesophagus, colon, rectum, lung, and in some types of breast cancer.

An authoritative review of the role of PSK in cancer concluded that:

"While PSK is not a panacea for cancers, it can improve five year survival in some indications [patients] by as much as double" *(Alternative Medicine Review: Volume 5, Number 1, February 2000)*.

"Coriolus versicolor is one of the safest and most effective agents any doctor can use against chronic diseases"

At the Centrum Clinic in Amsterdam, complementary practitioners have specialised in treating patients with a variety of immune deficiency disorders, including HIV and AIDS, and cancer patients since 1984. *Coriolus versicolor* extract has recently been added to some treatment regimens.

Marijke Pfeiffer, a practitioner of Traditional Chinese Medicine at the clinic, says that an increase in white blood cell counts has been noted in the majority of patients treated with the extract *(Presentation by Ms. Marijke Pfeiffer, Centrum Integrale Geneeskunde, Amsterdam, at the Third Symposium on Mushroom Nutrition)*.

Dr Steven Bailey, a naturopathic doctor based in Portland, Oregon, has been using *Coriolos versicolur* extract since 1998 to successfully treat patients with hepatitis B and C, AIDS, herpes, and to assist post-surgical recovery.

His cancer patients undergoing radiotherapy or chemotherapy have also found great benefit in taking the mushroom extract, he says. Studies show that PSK seems to preserve immune system activity despite the immunosuppressive impact of radio- and chemotherapy.

"Of all medicinal plants, *Coriolus versicolor* is one of the safest and most effective agents any doctor can use against chronic diseases," Dr Bailey says. "This mushroom places no metabolic demand on the liver or extenuating stress on the kidneys."

What to take for maximum results

Whether you suffer from one of the ailments listed above, or are simply anxious to boost your immune system generally, *Coriolus versicolor* is definitely worth your consideration. Side effects are very rare but may include diarrhoea, vomiting, nausea, and skin pigmentation. Please consult with your doctor before taking *Coriolus versicolor*.

Each pill contains 500mg of *Coriolus versicolor* extract and the recommended dose is two to six tablets (depending on your requirements) daily with meals. Healthy people will see immune benefits on a dose of 1,000mg a day. For cancer patients, following surgery and during chemotherapy and radiotherapy, the recommended dose is 3,000mg daily. Obviously it should only be used in conjunction with these treatments with your doctor's prior knowledge.

- **The natural remedy that could soon break into the mainstream as a cancer treatment used alongside chemotherapy**

As mentioned many times already throughout *The Cancer Survival Manual – Tomorrow's Cancer Breakthroughs Today*, a strong immune system is the key to good health. Yet there are numerous risk factors – such as pollution, stress, poor diet, medicinal drugs and environmental toxins – that place a huge burden on your body and can weaken your immune system. It's hardly surprising given all these culprits that diseases like cancer are so rife.

One way to promote immunity and prevent disease that has been rigorously researched is with mushrooms, as seen in the previous section. A brand new supplement called Mushroom Antioxidant Complex has been launched that harnesses the power of various medicinal mushrooms – including *coriolus versicolor* and reishi (both featured already on pages 275 and 272), maitake, and shiitake – in one supplement.

The combined effect of these oriental mushrooms with more established Western plant extracts, provides possibly one of the best ever natural defences against disease, especially cancer.

The additional ingredients in Mushroom Antioxidant Complex include: citrus pectin (an extract from the peel and pulp of citrus fruit), indole-3-carbinol (found in broccoli), lutein (a carotenoid found in red peppers, spinach and egg yolk), acerola (cherry extract), quercetin (found in many fruits and vegetables) and beta-carotene (found in yellow and orange fruits and vegetables, such as carrots).

Conventional cancer treatments can leave your weakened immune system open to attack

Your immune system is made up of white blood cells, which destroy micro-organisms by engulfing them, and lymphocytes. There are two types of lymphocytes, known as B-cells and T-cells. The latter can destroy foreign bodies directly whereas B-cells produce antibodies to inactivate undesirable substances, such as bacteria and viruses.

Other cells, known as natural killer (NK) cells, directly attack and destroy cancer cells before they get a chance to grow. When working properly, these immune cells are on constant lookout for abnormal cells, which can replicate out of control and form a tumour.

Conventional treatments for cancer include surgery to remove the tumour and surrounding tissue. Chemotherapy – the use of selective chemicals to destroy cancer cells by impairing their ability to replicate – is commonly used too. However chemotherapy drugs are highly toxic and can cause immunosuppression – where the immune system is weakened and leaves the patient more susceptible to infection.

This treatment is often used in conjunction with radiation treatment, which targets cancer cells using X-rays or gamma rays to deter the spread of malignant cells. It can cause distressing symptoms such as nausea, vomiting and hair loss.

Mushrooms offer a successful, less aggressive approach to cancer management

According to a report from Cancer Research UK, medicinal mushrooms may herald the start of a new era of cancer treatment and prevention. The report contained the most comprehensive review of studies ever carried out into the use of medicinal mushrooms – including reishi, shiitake and maitake (all contained in Mushroom Antioxidant Complex) – and revealed how they can help reduce the side effects of radiation treatment and chemotherapy, and significantly improve the quality of life of patients with advanced cancer *(Cancer Research UK. Mushrooms may work wonders in cancer treatment prevention. Report 19/08/02).*

Dr Richard Sullivan, head of clinical programmes for Cancer Research UK, said: "A vast amount of information has been collated, which suggests that compounds derived from mushrooms could have a hugely beneficial influence on the way cancer is treated."

For example, maitake has been found to exert an anti-tumour effect in mice by boosting the immune system through the activation of cancer-fighting cells like T-cells and NK cells. When Japanese researchers at Kobe Pharmaceutical University gave maitake extract to cancer patients, who were not being treated with anti-cancer drugs, they found that NK cell activity was significantly increased *(J Med Food 2003 Winter; 6(4): 371-7).*

In a separate study, the same researchers observed cancer regression or significant symptom improvement in 58.3 per cent of liver cancer patients, 68.8 per cent of breast cancer patients and 62.5 per cent of lung cancer patients. Maitake was also found to enhance the effectiveness of chemotherapy in the patients involved in this study *(Altern. Med Rev. 2002 Jun; 7(3): 236-9)*.

Other mushrooms in the formula also have a wide range of health benefits

As mentioned on pages 81 and 272, the reishi mushroom (present in Mushroom Antioxidant Complex) is known as the 'plant of immortality' in Traditional Chinese Medicine, as it is thought to promote longevity and fight cancer. It has been shown to possess anti-tumour, anti-inflammatory, and antiviral properties *(Chilton JS (1994). The first international conference on mushroom biology and mushroom products. Herbalgram 31:57; Amer.J. Chin. Med. 21:59-69); (Kim, BK et al. Anti-HIV activities of ganoderma lucidum. From the fifth International Mycological Congress Abstracts. Vancouver, BC August 1994.14-12)*.

The shiitake mushroom has also been credited with having anti-tumour activities, and researchers at the National University of Singapore have found that it can reduce the size of colon tumours in mice *(J Alt. Complement Med. 2002 Oct; 8(5): 581-9)*.

Even people without cancer can benefit from mushroom therapy. In a recent study, researchers at the Chinese University of Hong Kong studied the effects of *Coriolus versicolor* on the immune systems of 100 healthy subjects.

They found that regular oral consumption of the mushroom significantly increased immune cell counts, such as T-cells and NK cells. This suggests that mushroom therapy may have significant preventative properties, particularly beneficial to those at risk of immune-related diseases like cancer.

What to take for best results

The recommended dosage for Mushroom Antioxidant Complex is one to three capsules a day, or as otherwise recommended by your healthcare practitioner.

Contraindications: The Mushroom Antioxidant Complex is not recommended during pregnancy or breastfeeding. In addition, you should not take it if you are currently on warfarin, heparin, calcium channel blockers, the Pill, HRT or immune-suppressing medications.

• Could this overlooked 'waste product' be the cancer-fighting breakthrough of the century?

A new discovery is yielding results that are nothing short of astounding... tumour metastasis reduced by 82 per cent. A human study in which 31 per cent of cancer cells were flat out killed in 30 days. Oh, and the incredible results aren't just limited to cancer... sufferers of heart disease and enlarged prostates are also benefiting.

The source of this miracle cure? Flax. But, this isn't the same flax seed you've been used to seeing on your local health food store shelves. In fact, it's not flax seed at all.

The breakthrough that takes aim at cancer cells like a heat-seeking missile is Concentrated Flax Hull Lignans. They are concentrated directly – using a special process – from flax seed shells, or hulls, which typically don't make it into the bags of flax seed in the store. Which is a shame, because it turns out the vast majority of the disease-fighting lignans in the flax seed are located in the hull that encases the seed.

The nutrients contained in flax seeds are highly concentrated in the shells – one teaspoon of Concentrated Flax Hull Lignans contains the nutritional equivalent of two gallons of flax seed. Yes, gallons. And flax seed oil? Forget it. There are practically no lignans contained in the oil.

Lignans are a group of chemical compounds found in plants. They're one of the major classes of phytoestrogens, which are chemicals that act as antioxidants. Flax seed is the richest source of lignans in the plant kingdom, containing up to 800 times more than any other plant source. There are 27 different lignans in the flax seed and scientists believe they all work together to provide their amazing health benefits.

The major lignan in flax seed is called secoisolariciresinol diglucoside (SDG). It's actually a lignan precursor, which means its power isn't unlocked until it is metabolized by your body. In the intestines, SDG becomes two lignans. As we discovered in the course of our research, there's not much these lignans can't do when it comes to maintaining good health.

A new process unlocks this 'super food's' disease-fighting prowess

Though scientists have known for some time that the flax seed hulls have an amazing nutritional profile, they've been at a loss as to how to unlock those nutrients. Finally, a farmer by the name of Curtis Rangeloff invented a chemical-free method of mechanically separating the lignan-rich hulls from the rest of the flax.

Concentrated Flax Hull Lignans boast a pure lignan content of up to 65 per cent. Each scoop of the product contains 150-300mg of SDG per serving. That's 70 times the amount of SDG typically contained in the same amount of traditional ground flax seed.

In addition to their lignan content, flax seed hulls contain high levels of omega-3s, as well as off-the-charts antioxidants. To put it in perspective – kale has one of the highest ORAC values (a measurement of antioxidant content) at 1,770 per 100g. Concentrated Flax Hull Lignans? They come in at a whopping 19,600 per 100g. The hulls also contain 4.3g of fibre and 2.8g of protein in each tablespoon.

And while the nutritional value of Concentrated Flax Hull Lignans is certainly a bonus, the true value of the product is in its promise as a potent cancer-killer.

Driving cancer cells to 'mass suicide'

In two animal studies both breast tumour growth and metastasis were significantly reduced. In one of the studies, metastasis to the lungs was reduced by 82 per cent. The average number of tumours was also considerably lower in the test group than in the control group *(Nutr Cancer. 2002; 43(2): 187-92)*.

One of the most exciting cancer studies was carried out in Canada on a group of postmenopausal women with newly diagnosed breast cancer. Each day for a month, the women in the test group ate a flax seed muffin containing a predetermined concentration of SDG. After only one month, the growth of the cancer cells was reduced by 34.2 per cent. Even better, 31 per cent of cancer cells were completely killed, and the expression of the cancer growth receptor Her2 (c-erB2) – which causes tumours to grow more quickly and become more aggressive – decreased by 71 per cent *(Cancer Res. 2005 May 15; 11(10): 3828-35)*.

A study in California demonstrated that SDG reduced the risk of endometrial cancer in some women by 32 per cent. This reduced risk was most evident among postmenopausal women who consumed high levels of both isoflavones and lignans *(J Natl Cancer Inst. 2003; 95: 1158-1164)*. Other studies have shown similar reduced risk for uterine and ovarian cancers.

And, according to studies with human colon cancer cells, lignans stunt the growth of tumour cells and actually drive them to what can only be described as 'mass suicide' *(Journal of Nutrition. December 2006; 136: 3046-3053; Cancer Epidemiology Biomarkers and Prevention. August 2006; 15: 1555-1558)*.

Supplementation with SDG reduced tumours significantly in mice with melanoma. The average number of tumours in the control group was 62, while the average number in the groups of mice receiving SDG was around half that. Tumour size was also decreased *(Cancer Lett. 1999 July 19; 142(1): 91-6)*.

The scientific evidence doesn't stop at its cancer-fighting abilities...

In a 12-year study of Finnish men, it was found that those with the highest intake of plant lignans were significantly less likely to die from cardiovascular disease than their counterparts who ate the least amount of foods containing plant lignans *(Arch Intern Med. 2003; 163(9): 1099-1104)*.

Animal studies have shown that flax lignans can suppress the development of atherosclerosis (chronic inflammation of the arteries due to an accumulation of plaque) in addition to lowering cholesterol levels *(Atherosclerosis. 2005 April; 179(2): 269-275)*.

In a study involving Native American postmenopausal women, it was found that flax seed lowered LDL cholesterol by 10 per cent (*Womens Health. 2008 March 8. [Epub ahead of print]*). Mind you, that was just with flax seed, not the nutritionally-rich hulls.

Finally, no more late-night trips to the loo

A recent animal study demonstrated that flax lignans could also reduce prostate size. Rats given the human equivalent of 50mg per day of SDG (remember, Concentrated Flax Hull Lignans contain up to 300mg per serving) had significantly smaller prostates than those without the SDG supplementation. The SDG didn't just stop prostate growth – it actually helped reduce the size of the prostate *(Flax Lignan Information Bureau. 2005 May. http://www.flaxlignaninfo.com)*.

Lee, who describes himself as having a 'bad prostate,' has been using Concentrated Flax Hull Lignans for a couple of months. He has been making less and less trips to the toilet in the middle of the night, and says he generally feels better.

Though there are no conclusive studies concerning flax lignans and prostate cancer, there are a few that are promising. In a trial using mice, flax inhibited the growth and development of prostate cancer.

In a study of 25 men who were scheduled for prostatectomy, supplementation with flax brought significant changes in serum cholesterol, total testosterone, and the free androgen index. Researchers concluded that flax lignans may be a very beneficial food for men battling prostate cancer *(Urology. 2001; 58: 47–52)*.

Not only that but flax hull lignans can help boost immunity and are showing promise against both HIV and influenza *(AIDS Research Assistance Institute)*.

• How to overcome cancer-related fatigue

If you know someone who's struggling with cancer, one of the best gifts you could possibly give them is a tip on how to overcome fatigue.

Here's the tip: L-carnitine – a key amino acid produced in the kidneys and liver. Carnitine delivers fatty acids to cell mitochondria, helps protect cells (especially heart cells), raises the levels of certain enzymes needed to metabolize carbohydrates, and helps boost energy and muscle strength.

The body doesn't produce high levels of carnitine, but those levels are enhanced by dietary sources such as meat, chicken, fish, and dairy products. Unfortunately, the body only absorbs about a quarter of the carnitine supplied by food. And the problem is further complicated by the fact that our carnitine levels progressively decrease as we age.

Carnitine deficiency is known to be common among cancer patients. The primary trigger of this deficiency is chemotherapy, which blocks carnitine reabsorption by the kidneys. When carnitine levels drop, fatigue sets in – a challenging situation for cancer patients who may also suffer from anaemia and other energy-robbing problems related to their disease.

Researchers at Beth Israel Medical Center in New York City posed the question: Can carnitine supplements reduce fatigue in cancer patients with carnitine deficiency?

STUDY ABSTRACT

- Researchers recruited 27 patients with advanced cancer, carnitine deficiency, and moderate to severe fatigue.
- Before and after supplement intervention, subjects completed questionnaires to measure fatigue, depression, and quality of sleep.
- Subjects were divided into seven small groups to receive different daily doses of carnitine: 250mg, 750mg, 1,250mg, 1,750mg, 2,250mg, 2,750mg, and 3,000mg.
- The intervention period lasted seven days.
- Of the 21 patients who completed the study, 17 increased their carnitine levels.
- Overall, fatigue significantly decreased, while depression and sleep scores also improved.
- The most positive results were found among subjects who received the highest doses.
- Even at higher levels, the supplements were well tolerated.

Lead researcher, Dr Ricardo A Cruciani, told Reuters Health that a larger trial to test carnitine supplementation on a cohort of severely fatigued patients with cancer and other chronic diseases is about to get underway *(Journal of Pain and Symptom Management, Vol. 32, No. 6, December 2006).*

If you know someone who is coping with the debilitating effects of chronic fatigue, please pass this tip along. Of course, anyone who hopes to alleviate disease-related fatigue with L-carnitine supplements should first talk to their doctor.

- ## Chinese plant may help fight cancer and ageing as well as chronic diseases like arthritis and heart disease

Two and a half thousand years ago, Arab travellers trading with Chinese merchants came across an aromatic plant used both in cooking and as a health remedy. The Arabs were impressed by this plant which was used extensively by Chinese healers, so they introduced it to Europe where, over the centuries, it remained in obscurity until recently.

The plant is called *Cinnamomum cassia*, similar to cinnamon, but with a darker and thicker bark. Cassia is native to Burma, but it is grown across China, as well as in the West Indies, Indonesia, Australia and Central America *(J Ethnopharmacol 1991; 34(2-3): 173-87)*.

It's also known as 'bastard cinnamon', 'tejpat' or 'Chinese cinnamon'. It has a much stronger flavour compared to ordinary cinnamon, and it is used in stews and casseroles, curries, and spicy meat dishes.

Although cassia is still used as an aromatic herb today, its use in medicine was not widely appreciated by European health practitioners. However, recent research shows that cassia may have enormous potential for use as a health-boosting plant, particularly with regards to its antioxidant properties which are useful against cancer and other chronic diseases associated with ageing.

Has the potential to help get rid of cancerous cells before they can form a tumour

In China, cassia was traditionally used as a tonic and stimulant, and to improve bowel conditions such as diarrhoea, bloatedness, and nausea *(Food Chem Toxicol 1997; 35(6): 625-32)*. One of its main ingredients is the plant chemical called cinnamaldehyde.

This works in a variety of ways against cancer and age-related diseases. For example, research from the Kaohsiung Medical University in Taiwan shows that cinnamaldehyde is a strong chemical that may potentially help block cancer cells from developing, and assist the body in eliminating any abnormal or cancerous cells.

The scientists based their research on previous experiments which confirmed that cinnamaldehyde is effective at reducing the risk of cancer in humans. They wanted to investigate this further, and find out exactly how this ingredient of cassia may be able to block cancer.

What they discovered was that cinnamaldehyde helps activate several chemicals in the body (such as Bcl-2 and apoptotic factors) which may then speed up the elimination of cancerous cells before these can clump together and start a full-blown tumour *(Life Sci 2005; 77(8): 938-51)*.

In this way, cassia may prevent cancer from developing. It is not yet known whether cassia can help cure existing cancers but research in this field is continuing and new developments are due to be announced soon.

Conventional chemotherapy-boosting properties as well?

In addition to possibly being effective against cancer, cassia may help strengthen the activities of conventional anti-cancer drugs. Chinese doctors studied cassia as found in a traditional Chinese remedy called 'Shi-quan-da-bu-tang' (SQT), a well-known tonic used in oriental medicine (also containing herbal extracts from plants such as ginseng, astragalus and liquorice).

They reported that SQT helped boost the biological activities of drugs commonly used against cancer such as mitomycin, cisplatin, cyclophosphamide and fluorouracil. The researchers believe that: "SQT inhibits the recurrence of malignancies, prolongs survival, and prevents adverse side effects such as loss of appetite, nausea, vomiting, anaemia and kidney problems which are associated with the use of many anti-cancer drugs" *(Methods Find Exp Clin Pharmacol 1992, 14(9): 725-36).*

This may be an added bonus of cassia which means that it could be effective either on its own or in combination with strong drugs used in conventional chemotherapy.

Cassia has strong anti-free radical properties which may help fight against ageing and chronic diseases

In a different experiment, Italian scientists from the Department of Bio-organic Chemistry, University of Pisa, found that essential oil from cassia (which contains eugenol, thought to be a strong and beneficial ingredient of the bark) is powerful against free radicals.

These toxic by-products of your everyday metabolism have been linked not only to cancer but also to ageing and chronic diseases (such as arthritis, heart disease, dementia and cataract). If left uncontrolled, free radicals continue to develop until they cause what we call 'ageing'.

During the Italian experiment, the eugenol ingredient of cassia was found to block one particular free radical molecule called 'peroxynitrite', a very common and lethal chemical, found in all of us in small amounts. With the peroxynitrite molecules under control by eugenol, the body may then be able to function again at full strength, and the risk of cancer and ageing could be reduced *(J Agric Food*

Chem 2005; 53(12): 4762-5).

What to take for best results

The bark of cassia is available from Chinese food stores. The dose is 0.6g to 1.6g of powder daily. There are no reported contraindications. Cassia is recommended for Type 2 diabetics only, as it encourages the production of insulin. If you're currently taking medications for blood sugar, you should consult your doctor before trying this remedy.

• **Perillyl alcohol – a natural compound found in cherries may help fight cancer**

Although they are small, tart cherries pack quite a healthy punch. They contain over 17 natural compounds that work synergistically to promote a healthy body. And now a concentrated form is available that gives you the benefit of the whole cherry in a much more convenient capsule called Fruit Advantage Tart Cherry Capsules.

Not only is the tart cherry a potent antioxidant, it also contains high concentrations of a compound that appears to have the potential to help prevent, stabilize and possibly eliminate cancer... although more research is needed to confirm initial findings.

According to Dr Raymond Hohl, at the University of Iowa, a natural compound found in tart cherries – perillyl alcohol (POH) – "shuts down the growth of cancer cells by depriving them of the proteins they need to grow." He went on to say that: "It works on every kind of cancer we've tested it against."

The new star in anti-cancer research

The tart cherry is quickly becoming the star of POH research, although smaller levels of POH have also been found in the essential oils of lavender, peppermint, sage and lemon grass. POH is a member of a new class of anti-cancer agents called monoterpenes.

Monoterpenes are found in the highly concentrated volatile, aromatic essences of plants – the essential oils. They're formed in the mevalonic pathway in plants – the same pathway that makes cholesterol in animals and humans.

Early on, researchers realised that some aspects of cholesterol metabolism were involved in cancer growth: This pathway appears to affect rapid cell growth called proliferation *(J Nutr 1994; 124: 607-14)*.

Then they discovered that plant monoterpenes not only interfered with animal cholesterol synthesis and reduced animals' cholesterol levels, but that they also reduced tumour formation in the animals by helping to halt proliferation *(Biochim Biophys Acta 1999; 1,449(2): 137-149)*.

With this new awareness researchers began to focus on two specific monoterpenes – limonene and POH. When they compared the two, their studies showed that POH was five times as active in regressing tumours as limonene *(Crowell PL, et al. "Antitumor effects of limonene and perillyl alcohol against pancreatic and breast cancer." Dietary Phytochemicals in Cancer Prevention and Treatment. New York: Plenum Press, 1996; Cancer Lett 1995; 96: 15-21)*. The exact actions of monoterpenes is still unknown, but POH's ability to block the pathway leading to cell proliferation might explain it.

When the DNA in a human cell becomes damaged, the cell malfunctions. Its growth goes unregulated, and if this cell isn't capable of initiating its natural self-destruction sequence (apoptosis), the result is often cancerous growth. It appears that POH might step in and regulate the growth and apoptosis processes that the malfunctioning cell can't.

This idea is backed-up by several animal trials, where POH has been shown to prevent carcinogenesis, the process by which normal cells are transformed into cancer cells. POH has shown chemopreventive activity in liver cancer in rats, pancreatic cancer in hamsters, non-melanoma skin cancer in mice, and breast cancer in rats *(Cancer Res 1995; 55: 979-83; Cancer Lett 1995; 96: 15-21; Cancer Res 1998; 58: 711-16; Cancer Chemother Pharmacol 1994; 34: 477-83).*

And the percentages are nothing to brush off. Take the last example – breast cancer in rats – where POH slowed the growth of 81 per cent of small tumours and up to 75 per cent of advanced tumours.

Human trials have also had some encouraging results. In one National Cancer Institute-sponsored trial performed at the University of Wisconsin, Madison, in the US, researchers found evidence that POH may slow or even reverse the progression of colorectal cancer *(Clin Cancer Res 2000; 6: 390-96).*

In the human trials, there does seem to be one problem, in the form of stomach upset. Although some researchers felt that the soya used in the original POH test formula may be the real cause. When they varied the formula and participants took it with food the results were better. Andy LaPointe, CEO and founder of FruitCeuticals, who manufacture Fruit Advantage Tart Cherry Capsules, was asked if he'd had any similar feedback regarding stomach upset. He said he hadn't. In fact, there haven't been any reports of side effects.

Get your share of the antioxidant goldmine's 'mother lode'

LaPointe claims that one of the major benefits his product offers over other cherry products is that the whole cherry is used – even the skin. Many liquid cherry concentrations discard this part of the fruit, but, in fact, it's the skin that contains the beneficial anthocyanins, which LaPointe described as the potential "mother lode in a goldmine of antioxidants."

Anthocyanins are naturally occurring compounds that impart colour to fruit, vegetables and plants. They are thought to play a major role in the high antioxidant activity levels observed in red and blue fruits and vegetables.

In the manufacturing process, the stem and the pit are removed, then the cherries are dried, ground up, and put in a vegetarian capsule.

LaPointe was careful to point out that Fruit Advantage Tart Cherry Capsules are really intended for use as a daily supplement to assist with overall maintenance of a healthy body. But the promising research emerging about POH's potential role as an anti-cancer agent makes this product an exciting find *(J Pharmacol Exp Ther 2004; 311(2): 568-75)*.

Get the benefits of cherries now – even before the proof is 'official'

'More research needed' is the recurring theme when it comes to tart cherries' benefits. Although the initial studies' results look promising, keep in mind that as far as POH in cancer treatment goes, this application is still being researched.

But one thing is certain: knowing the potential of POH in tart cherries may put you ahead of the curve and enable you to get all these potential benefits just by using it as a daily supplement.

What to take for best results

Fruit Advantage Tart Cherry Capsules provide 850mg of the whole Montmorency tart cherries. The suggested daily dose is two capsules per day. While no side effects were reported from users of the Fruit Advantage Tart Cherry Capsules, in human trials some patients taking POH did report stomach upset.

• Discover the plant extract that is proving invaluable in the fight against cancer

Elecampane *(Inula helenium)* is a perennial plant that grows throughout Europe and Asia and produces distinct yellow spiky flowers... which is how it gained its nickname 'wild sunflower'.

It has been used in folk medicine for thousands of years and was prized by ancient Greek healers as an effective remedy for the treatment of respiratory problems like coughs, bronchitis and emphysema.

It is still used for this purpose today. The dried plant roots and rhizomes (branching part of the root) are collected in the spring or early winter, as they are a rich source of volatile oils that act as an expectorant – helping to clear the lungs of any phlegm. In addition, the root extract contains inulin – a natural chemical, which soothes and relaxes the lungs.

Elecampane is a beneficial treatment for numerous other disorders including diabetes, circulation problems, joint pains, indigestion and the common cold (by promoting perspiration). It is also an effective tonic that promotes overall well-being. On top of that it is showing promise in the fight against cancer too...

Root extract helps defend against harmful free radicals

Japanese scientists from the Faculty of Pharmaceutical Sciences, at the University of Tokushima, examined several Asian herbs, including Elecampane, for their ability to reduce levels of harmful free radicals such as nitric oxide and oxygen peroxide.

Free radicals are dangerous chemicals that are implicated in causing numerous serious conditions, including cancer, and are produced by your cells following exposure to pollution, cigarette smoke, alcohol and stress.

When the scientists studied elecampane they discovered that it contains several hitherto unknown chemicals – variants of sesquiterpene lactones – that have turned out to be powerful antioxidants that can neutralise harmful free radicals (*Phytomedicine. 2004 Nov; 11(7-8): 645-51*).

More evidence to support the theory that elecampane may play an important role in the fight against cancer has come from additional research conducted in Japan. Doctors studying the effects of the root extract found that several types of cancer cells – including those of the liver, lung and skin – were killed by the extract. They believe that certain types of sesquiterpenes – such as germacrane and alantolactone – present in the root, are responsible for this anti-cancer action *(Biol Pharm Bull. 2002 Oct; 25(10): 1370-2).*

What to take for best results

The recommended dosage for elecampane root is two capsules (each containing 503mg of elecampane root) taken three times a day with water – or as otherwise directed on the product's label.

It is important that you consult your doctor first before taking the herb, especially if you are currently on any medication.

Contraindications: Pregnant and breast-feeding women should not use elecampane.

- ### Graviola: This Amazonian remedy provides potent anti-cancer benefits

The shameless greed of a major drug company, who covered up news of an extraordinary cancer-fighter called graviola just because it couldn't figure out a way to profit from the discovery, is truly shocking.

If it wasn't for the fateful conversation between a secret insider and one brave woman, the world might never have learned about this astounding breakthrough.

Enter Leslie Taylor – a modern jungle-trekking medicine woman who spends most of her days in the company of Amazonian tribes. She soaks up their generations-old wisdom so she can share their secrets.

She was a key player in the graviola exposé. When a confidential source with access to graviola's secret studies buckled under the weight of his conscience, he contacted Taylor with the truth about the tree's healing properties.

Digging deeper, she discovered that there was a small body of published research that corroborated these conclusions. So she put together a harvesting operation, manned by indigenous South American tribes, to collect graviola's potent leaves and stems and formulate them into a cancer-fighting remedy.

Graviola has been the subject of dozens of published studies touting its unmatched power against a whole army of cancers, including liver, lung, breast, skin, kidney, prostate and colon… just to name a few.

But Taylor's research continued and this recently led to another form of graviola being uncovered – one that's taking the original's tumour-fighting properties to a whole new level.

A new tropical tree introduces 26 additional cancer-fighting chemicals

Mountain graviola is a new species of the genus Annona, the active compounds of which are called acetogenins – and Taylor discovered it herself during a visit to her South American harvesting site.

Though strikingly similar in appearance to the original species of graviola (also known as *Annona muricata*), she noticed that natives never ate the fruit of this new tree – while the fruit, stems, and leaves of its close relative were regularly consumed by local tribes for medicinal purposes. After questioning them as to the reason, she was told that, unlike graviola, the fruit from the mountain graviola tree (or *Annona montana*) was far too sour to be edible.

But a closer look at the plant's structure revealed that this substitution had been coming at a price. Although the sweeter graviola does in fact deliver potent therapeutic properties, the less-palatable mountain graviola has nearly 26 novel acetogenins that you won't find in its relative – and even more of the acetogenin annonacin, which has been the focus of most of the published studies on account of its demonstrated cancer-fighting abilities and lack of toxicity.

Unlike its counterpart *Annona muricata*, research on the specific components of mountain graviola has only begun to pick up in the last few years.

Mountain graviola could herald a breakthrough in the fight against ovarian and liver cancer

Japanese scientists are credited with detecting unique acetogenins in mountain graviola and testing them against lung cancer cell lines. For research purposes they used the chemotherapy drug Andriamycin as a control. Results showed that several of these isolated compounds (with a specific focus on the acetogenin montanacin) demonstrated an ability to inhibit tumour growth that was comparable to the actions of the powerful, but very toxic, chemotherapy drug *(Bioorg. Med. Chem. 2002; 10(3): 561-5; Planta Med. 2001 Dec; 67(9): 807-11).*

Additional compelling evidence has revealed mountain graviola's cancer-fighting properties against liver and ovarian cancer. In one study a range of nine new acetogenins present in mountain graviola were tested. Findings demonstrated that the isolated compounds acted selectively against the human ovarian cancer line 1A9 and liver cancer Hep G2 cells *(Planta Med. 2004 Oct; 70(10): 948-59).*

This study was closely followed by further research which tested two of these new acetogenins (montacin and cis-montacin) along with four already-known acetogenins. Results further confirmed that the new compounds are able to prevent the spread of human ovarian cancer cells *(J Nat Prod. 2004 Nov; 67(11): 1804-8).*

In another more recent study, two types of acetogenins were isolated from mountain graviola and were again subjected to a cytotoxicity test against eight human cancer cell lines. While select compounds demonstrated moderate cytotoxic activities against six of these cancerous cell lines (including lung), all of the compounds once again showed significantly more powerful activity when pitted against ovarian and liver cancer cell lines *(Bioorg. Med. Chem. 2005 Aug 1; 13 (15): 4767-76).*

New, super-strength combo helps combat deadly cancers

While no clinical trials have been conducted as yet for either graviola or mountain graviola, Taylor has received numerous testimonials – many from customers who had been using a new, super-strength proprietary blend of both forms of graviola, which delivers a total of 108 documented cancer-fighting acetogenins. It's called Graviola Max by Raintree Nutrition.

One woman, who was diagnosed with colon cancer for the second time in May of 2006, opted against chemotherapy after her tumour was surgically removed – choosing instead to begin a rigorous regimen of supplementation with both Graviola Max and N-Tense. According to her husband, her report seven months later was extremely encouraging, with all indicators pointing to what appears to be a full remission.

"I can truthfully say that had I not begun to use Graviola, I most likely would not be alive today," began the striking testimonial of another woman, who was diagnosed with oesophageal cancer in January 2006. At the time of her diagnosis, she had been unable to consume anything but liquids.

She began supplementing with the product during her chemotherapy and radiation visits – eight months later, she was in complete remission, and able to eat solid foods once again. Today, she's cancer-free, and continues to supplement with Graviola Max.

Though it might be a while before we're actually able to see the long-term results of treatment with Graviola Max, these initial reports are more than promising. And when combined with the incredible stories of recovery from longtime graviola users, these accounts add an entirely new dimension to the already compelling laboratory research findings.

What to take for best results

Because Graviola Max is so strong, it's not recommended for use as a preventative. Take three capsules three to four times a day, or as otherwise directed by your healthcare practitioner. You should be aware that a common side effect is nausea – resulting from the products main cancer-fighting ingredient, annonacin.

Taylor has also developed a new tincture called Stomach-Ez (made from the extracts of a variety of South American tropical plants) to help eliminate any queasiness or vomiting that might result from supplementation with Graviola Max.

- **Discover the superior form of cat's claw that defends against disease by protecting and repairing your body's precious DNA**

Cat's claw *(Uncaria tomentosa)* is a giant woody vine that grows in the Amazon rainforest and has been treasured for its medicinal properties for over 2,000 years. The native Indians of South America used it to heal all manner of ailments, from rheumatism and arthritis, to dysentery, gastric ulcers and even tumours. Since the early 1990s it has also been used as a natural remedy in both Peru and Europe for strengthening the immune system and relieving inflammation.

Most commercial cat's claw products are simply, dried ground herbal powder. However, a new generation of the herb has become available that is prepared according to the traditional method of hot water extraction, making the active components more bioavailable and better able to maintain good health.

Known as AC-11, the process used to produce cat's claw in this form not only provides superior bioavailability, but isolates potent carboxy alkyl esters (CAEs) – the active constituents in the plant. In addition, hot water extraction helps eliminate potentially irritating compounds called oxindole alkaloids, that can cause cramping and diarrhoea in sensitive people.

Although research has demonstrated that cat's claw is a potent anti-inflammatory and immune enhancer, only AC-11 has been shown in scientific studies to protect and repair vital DNA. This is a major breakthrough as DNA repair can lead to strengthened immunity, the prevention of chronic diseases, such as cancer, and even a reversal of the ageing process.

How DNA affects your overall health and well-being

DNA (deoxyribonucleic acid) is a nucleic acid within every human cell that carries important genetic information needed to construct and maintain your body. It is often compared to an individual's blueprint for life.

Consisting of two long strands of nucleotides twisted into a double helix, the sequence of nucleotides determines your individual hereditary characteristics. When cells divide creating new ones to replace the old, DNA is replicated so that each new cell has an exact copy of the blueprint or genetic information.

Every day the DNA in your cells is constantly being attacked by free radicals – unstable and highly reactive molecules which accelerate the progression of age-related diseases. While antioxidant compounds such as vitamin C and selenium are able to protect your DNA by neutralising free radicals, they are powerless to help fix the damage once it has occurred.

Once DNA has been attacked, its strands become pitted. Sometimes a strand may break, and occasionally double-strand breaks occur. These are the most serious types of breaks, as when cells divide creating new ones, these new cells will get an altered blueprint. Taking it one step further, as cells continue to divide, your body will keep on making poor copies of copies, and as DNA degradation gets worse this has a detrimental effect on your overall health and longevity.

Fortunately, your body has an innate ability to repair altered DNA and this complex repairing process takes place thousands of times a day. However, sometimes the rate of DNA attack can outpace the rate of DNA repair – unrepaired DNA damage being the basis for ageing and disease.

AC-11 is one of the best researched compounds available that helps repair damaged DNA, and so far is the only natural agent known with this ability. As an antioxidant, it also prevents DNA from being damaged in the first place.

Studies reveal AC-11's remarkable ability to repair damaged DNA

In a laboratory study, AC-11 was tested for its ability to modulate DNA repair in human skin organ cultures. The skin cultures were pre-treated topically with AC-11 before being exposed to various levels of UV radiation. They were then treated with the active compound again. AC-11 was shown to enhance sunlight protection and significantly increase DNA repair *(Phytother Res. 2006; 20(3): 178-83).*

In another study, AC-11 was tested in humans for its DNA repairing efficiency. After eight weeks of supplementation, the participants showed a significant increase in the ability to repair DNA – about 12 to 15 per cent – following a dose of free radical producing hydrogen peroxide *(Phytomedicine 2001; 8: 275-282).*

In a further study, the effectiveness of a broad spectrum antioxidant supplement with and without the addition of AC-11 was compared. Healthy individuals were divided into two groups. Group one received the antioxidant formula alone, while group two received the antioxidants plus AC-11.

Results showed that both the antioxidants alone and the antioxidants combined with AC-11 were effective anti-ageing interventions. However, the beneficial effects were far more pronounced when the two products were taken together – the antioxidant reduced DNA damage and AC-11 prevented an accumulation of damaged DNA and enhanced DNA repair *(Journal of Anti-aging Medicine 2002: 5: 345-353).*

AC-11 helps ward off everything from cancer to the common cold

Marcia Zimmerman, CN, one of the health industry's most well respected nutrition education specialists and author of *Reverse Ageing* (Nutrition Solution Publications), writes: "AC-11 is an antioxidant that prevents DNA damage. While this is extremely important, the story gets even better. AC-11 induces apoptosis (programmed cell death) and this enhances immune function, decreases inflammation, and kills tumour cells. Other nutritional agents share some of these activities. However, only AC-11 is a powerful enhancer of DNA repair and is the only natural agent known to do so."

AC-11 is ideal for anyone wanting to slow down the ageing process, improve skin quality and reduce the risk of degenerative diseases, particularly if there is a family history of cancer, heart disease, diabetes or other ageing conditions.

As an effective anti-inflammatory agent, AC-11 is able to help combat arthritis and other inflammatory diseases, such as cancer, in addition to enhancing the healing process following surgery. Its ability to reduce inflammation appears to work by negating the activation of NF-kappa B – a transcription factor that controls the production of pro-inflammatory cytokines.

The immune-enhancing effects of AC-11 make it particularly effective for general immune deficiency and preventing colds and flu.

What to take for best results

The recommended dosage for AC-11 is one capsule taken daily between meals. AC-11 is safe to take alongside most medications, although as a precaution anyone taking prescription drugs for a health condition should check with their GP before use. The product is best avoided during pregnancy and while breastfeeding.

Chapter Thirteen:
Much-needed relief from cancer pain

There are many different forms of pain relief available to cancer sufferers... meaning you needn't suffer unnecessarily. About one-third of all cancer patients experience pain, which can take many different forms. The two main ones include:

1. Pain from the tumour – most cancer pain arises when a tumour presses on bone, nerves or body organs. The pain may vary according to location. For example, a small tumour located near a nerve or the spinal cord may be very painful, while a larger tumour located elsewhere may not cause the patient any discomfort. It's important to bear in mind that pain does not always indicate tumour progression or recurrence.

In such cases an operation to remove all or part of the tumour may be all that is needed to provide relief from pain. Radiation therapy, which reduces pain by shrinking a tumour, can also help.

2. Pain related to cancer therapy. Chemotherapy, radiotherapy and surgery can all be painful. In addition, certain painful conditions are more likely to develop in patients with a suppressed immune system, which often results from these therapies.

The good news is that cancer pain is treatable and in the 21st century it is no longer necessary for patients to endure endless amounts of suffering. Although pain caused by the disease is usually treated with drugs, complementary treatments such as relaxation, hypnotherapy, TENS, biofeedback, massage and visualisation can also help.

It is important to be aware that complementary treatments should not be used as a substitute for your medicine, and it is important that you discuss their use with your doctor prior to trying them.

By using a combination of conventional and complementary therapies, you can help give your body a rest from pain, which can in turn aid your recovery... even to the extent that appetite and sleep normally improve when cancer-related pain is under control.

- ## Hypnotherapy – tap into the power of suggestion to overcome discomfort

Hypnosis is a state of altered awareness, which allows the person being hypnotized to become absorbed in more relaxing thoughts, ideas, images and feelings, and more easily distracted from negative or painful ones. Many people who benefit from hypnosis respond well to suggestions about feeling less pain, more comfort, increased energy, better sleep, and having rapid healing outcomes.

Hypnotic intervention has been used successfully for many types of specific pain. With cancer patients, hypnotic suggestion can help to reduce the suffering related to many painful procedures such as the administration of chemotherapy and treatment-related throat pain and nausea.

- ## Visualisation – picture yourself healthy, happy and pain free

Mind and emotions have been shown to be as important in the effective treatment of cancer as treating the body – and may be even more so. Visualisation can be an important tool for cancer patients to help overcome pain.

Visualisation is the technique of using the power of the mind – specifically the imagination – to help the body. It has been found to be effective in the treatment of a wide range of pain-related conditions – from back strain to cancer. In the case of cancer, sufferers are encouraged to visualise an army of healthy cells destroying all the cancer cells and replacing them with undamaged, healthy cells.

Visualisation seems to be particularly beneficial for people who are able to harness their imaginations at will. It is not known exactly how visualisation works in the management of pain, but the power of the mind to influence the body is clearly at the root of the process.

As an example, try imagining yourself in a place you know, where you feel happy, peaceful and content – you may find it easier to do this with your eyes closed and concentrating on regulating your breathing first. This could be a favourite place you remember from childhood like a lake or a forest that you visited on a family holiday, for instance. Gradually become part of the scene. Use all your senses – for example, try and recapture the smells and sounds around you. Visualise yourself feeling happy and healthy and completely pain free. Repeat this exercise on a regular basis and see if there is any change in your symptoms.

• Herbal pain relief

In addition, there are a wide range of herbs that can help alleviate pain caused by the disease – obviously these depend entirely on the symptoms and the individual, and it is vital that you work with a qualified medical herbalist (who works in conjunction with your doctor) to determine this. Common herbs used to relieve cancer pain include Jamaican dogwood, lady's slipper, passion flower, skullcap and valerian.

Homeopathic treatment with Nux vomica (3c or 6c, taken three times daily for a month) has been found to be effective for alleviating discomfort – particularly nausea – caused by conventional cancer treatments. Again, make sure you work closely with a qualified homeopath and your doctor.

• Herbal protection for chemo and radiation-therapy dangers

Ashwagandha, also known as 'winter cherry' and 'Indian ginseng', is a shrub found primarily in western India and Israel which has existed for 2,500 years. It has been used in Ayurvedic medicine to treat a variety of diseases, with its roots and leaves usually prepared as powders, oils and poultices.

Although ashwagandha is primarily known as an aphrodisiac, it also acts as a folk remedy against arthritis, asthma, colds, diarrhoea, fever, hiccups, hypertension, heart problems, inflammations, lumbago, nausea, psoriasis, rheumatism, ringworm, scabies, senility and syphilis.

Ashwagandha's effectiveness isn't restricted to protecting the immune system; it has also been shown to have anti-tumour effects.

Researchers from Banaras Hindu University in Varanasi, India, discovered that some of the chemicals in ashwagandha are very powerful antioxidants. They tested these for their effects on the brains of rats and found an increase in the levels of three natural antioxidants. This may explain the brain-strengthening, anti-stress, anti-inflammatory, and anti-ageing effects produced by the herb *(Indian J Physiol 41(4): 424-426, 1997)*.

There is evidence that ashwagandha aids radiation therapy and chemotherapy in the treatment of cancer. It appears to make the tumour more sensitive to radiation – thereby making it more vulnerable to radiation treatment. This was confirmed in studies conducted in 1993 and 1996 *(Indian J Exp Biol 31(7): 607-611, 1993; Indian J Exp Biol 34(10): 927-932, 1996)*.

One of the chief side effects of chemotherapy is immuno-suppression – the weakening of the body's natural defence against disease and infection. Leukopenia (an abnormal decrease in protective white blood cells) and myelosuppression (the acute weakening of bone marrow) are two manifestations of this immune-system breakdown.

A 1994 study showed that ashwagandha prevented both leukopenia and myelosuppression in animals treated with a chemotherapeutic chemical *(Tumori 80(4): 306-308, 1994)*. This result was repeated two years later, when the herb prevented myelosuppression in mice given three different immunosuppressive drugs *(J Ethnopharmacol 50(2): 69-76, 1996)*.

In a related effect, ashwagandha prolonged the survival of mice infected with aspergillus – a fungal infection/colonisation of the lung, sometimes brought on by the immunosuppressive effects of chemotherapy *(Immunopharmacol Immunotoxicol 20(1): 191-198, 1998)*.

A 1992 study found that doses of 400mg/kg given to mice with transplanted tumours "produced complete regression of tumour after an initial growth, the percentage of complete response increasing with increasing dose" *(Indian J Exp Biol 30(3): 169-172, 1992)*.

If you're facing the prospect of chemo or radiation therapy, ashwagandha might be an ally you could use in your corner.

- **Zyflamend's remarkable pain-relieving and inflammation fighting properties can help cancer patients**

Research has revealed that natural alternatives can successfully banish pain without causing any adverse effects like conventional painkillers. Ten herbs that have been found to be particularly beneficial in this area are holy basil, turmeric, ginger, green tea, rosemary, hu zhang, Chinese goldthread, barberry, oregano and scutellaria.

Now, following extensive research into their individual pain-relieving properties, these 10 herbs have been combined into a new formula called Zyflamend. It has been found to offer effective relief against pain caused by inflammatory conditions such as cancer and arthritis.

Zyflamend helps put the brakes on a pain-causing mechanism in your body

Zyflamend works in a similar way to NSAIDs, killing pain by decreasing the production of pro-inflammatory prostaglandins (hormone-like substances), which are generated by the cyclooxygenase (COX) enzyme.

There are in fact two cyclooxygenase enzymes – cyclooxygenase-1 (COX-1) and cyclooxygenase-2 (COX-2). COX-1 has many important functions in your cells and is continually being produced by your body. These functions include regulation of blood flow, platelet function, gastrointestinal protection and regulation of kidney function.

However, while the correct amount of COX-2 in the body is also vital for a number of biological functions, if its activity increases (often caused by an excess consumption of red meat, saturated fats and refined vegetable oils) so too does the presence of pain and inflammation.

Like NSAIDs, Zyflamend works by suppressing the effect of COX-2. Not only does this help control pain but there is also mounting evidence to suggest that this action may even protect against cancer, as raised COX-2 activity appears to increase the incidence of cancer.

For example, a number of studies have found elevated levels of COX-2 in prostate cancer cells (*Natural cyclooxygenase inhibitors and their potential activities against prostate cancer, Columbia-Presbyterian Medical Center, Summer 2002*). In addition, COX-2 is 60 times more prevalent in a cancerous pancreas than in a normal one and the enzyme may be present in up to 90 per cent of patients suffering from rectal cancer (*Dr James Duke, The most important medicine you'll ever grow: COX-2 inhibitors can ease pain and fight cancer – naturally. Special report Natural Health, part two*).

How the 10 herbs in Zyflamend work to combat pain and inflammation

The individual herbs contained in Zyflamend have each been extensively studied for their pain-relieving properties and potential anti-cancer activity. They include:

1. Holy basil. Indigenous to India, holy basil (not to be confused with common basil that is used as a culinary herb) contains ursolic acid. Research carried out at Dartmouth Medical School suggests that a strong link exists between ursolic acid's anti-inflammatory and anti-cancer actions and its ability to inhibit COX-2 *(Cancer Res 1998; 58(4): 717-23)*. In another study conducted in France, ursolic acid was recognised by scientists as, "a causative agent in the 'programmed' cell death of human leukaemia cells" *(FEBS Lett 1992; 299(3): 213-7)*.

2. Turmeric. The active constituent of turmeric, a common ingredient added to curries, is a plant chemical called curcumin. It has been shown to reduce inflammation by lowering histamine levels and preventing the overproduction of COX-2. Researchers conducting a preliminary trial involving rheumatoid arthritis patients found that curcumin was beneficial in reducing inflammation, pain and stiffness *(Ind J Med Res 1980; 71:632–4)*. A separate double-blind trial revealed that curcumin was superior to both placebo and phenylbutazone (a NSAID) for alleviating post-surgical inflammation and pain *(Int J Clin Pharmacol Ther Toxicol 1986; 24: 651–4)*.

3. Ginger also inhibits the COX-2 enzyme. According to authors Thomas M Newmark (medical researcher and writer) and Paul Schulick (herbalist, researcher and lecturer) of *Beyond Aspirin* (HOHM Press, 2000), "ginger not only safely modulates COX-2, but it also safely brings balance to COX-1 enzyme activity in a manner that is vastly superior to the synthetic NSAIDs, like aspirin."

4. Green Tea contains the potent COX-2 inhibitors salicylic acid and polyphenols. A 1999 study published in the US Government's Proceedings of the National Academy of Science refers to the polyphenols in green tea as having a "marked reduction" on COX-2 induced arthritis *(Proc Natl Acad Sci USA 1999; 96(8): 4524-9)*. Several experiments also suggest that the polyphenols it contains possess potent anti-cancer properties, particularly in terms of cancers of the stomach, small intestine, pancreas, colon, lung and breast *(Toxicol Sci 1999; 52(2 Suppl): 111–7; World Rev Nutr Diet 1996; 79:154–84 [review]; Nutr Cancer 1997; 27: 1–13 [review])*.

5. Rosemary. In 1998, Swedish scientists identified the COX-2 inhibiter ursolic acid in rosemary. It also contains apigenin, which researchers at the National University of Taiwan claim to be a "markedly active inhibitor of COX-2".

6. Hu zhang *(Polygonum cuspidatum)*. This herb, which is native to Japan, is the richest known source of a polyphenol called resveratrol, which acts as a powerful antioxidant and inhibitor of COX-2 *(Thomas M Newmark and Paul Schulick, Beyond Aspirin, HOHM Press 2000)*.

7 & 8. Chinese goldthread and Barberry both contain a compound called berberine that prevents excess amounts of COX-2. Besides its anti-inflammatory and anti-microbial properties, berberine has also been shown to exert an anti-cancer action in a number of studies *(J Ethnopharmacol 1999; 66(2): 227-33)*.

9. Oregano contains four compounds – apigenin, kaempherol, ursolic acid and oleanolic acid – that have displayed COX-2 inhibiting effects.

10. Scutellaria, also known as baikal skullcap, contains the flavonoid baicalein which suppresses COX-2. Korean scientists have found that scutellaria stimulates an important cancer detoxification enzyme called quinone reductase *(Eur J Cancer Prev 1998; 7(6): 465-71).* In addition, researchers in Japan have demonstrated that scutellaria is able to inhibit the spread of colon cancer *(Boil Pharm Bull 1998; 21(8): 814-7).*

Zyflamend encourages the destruction of cancerous cells

Laboratory tests conducted at the Center for Holistic Urology, Department of Urology, Columbia University in New York, and led by scientists Debra Bemis, PhD and Aaron Katz, MD, found that Zyflamend (which contains all of the 10 herbs mentioned above) slowed the growth of prostate cancer cells *(Bemis DL, Katz AE et al. Zyflamend, An herbal COX-2 inhibitor with in vitro anti-prostate-cancer activity. Center for Holistic Urology, Department of Urology, Columbia University, New York).*

In addition, Zyflamend also doubled the rate at which the cancerous cells self-destructed, a natural anti-cancer activity known as apoptosis or programmed cell death.

What to take for best results

The recommended dosage is one Zyflamend capsule taken twice a day with your main meal and with a glass of water.

WARNING: Women who are pregnant or trying for a baby should consult their GP before taking Zyflamend.

A final word of advice

One in three people will be affected by cancer at some stage in their life, so it's vital you take steps right now to reduce your risk. Instead of living in fear of becoming yet another cancer victim statistic, remember that 85 per cent of adult cancers are entirely avoidable according to the World Health Organsiation (WHO) and, of these, around half are related to nutritional deficiencies in the Western diet.

Having read *The Cancer Survival Manual – Tomorrow's Cancer Breakthroughs TODAY* you'll now know exactly what specific foods to eat more of and, just as importantly, those to avoid, in order to reduce your risk of succumbing to the disease.

We can't emphasize enough how making simple changes to your lifestyle – such as taking regular exercise, eating healthily, avoiding smoking and reducing your alcohol intake – can really pay off and dramatically reduce your cancer risk.

If you or a loved one is battling cancer it is important to remain as positive as possible. With the information contained in this book you'll be better placed to make informed decisions regarding your treatment options. You'll also know what dietary and lifestyle choices can help you recover.

According to data from the National Cancer Intelligence Network the number of cancer survivors could double in 20 years in Britain if rates continue to improve *(The Times 21/06/2010)*. Their findings revealed that across the UK, women with breast cancer and men with prostate cancer were most likely to survive for at least 10 years after having the disease; but the figures confirm the poor prognosis of lung cancer, survivors of which account for just three per cent of all cancer patients alive after 10 years. With regards to lung cancer, survival rates improve dramatically with early detection. After reading *The Cancer*

Survival Manual – Tomorrow's Cancer Breakthroughs TODAY you know the warning signs to look out for and the steps to take that can help prevent this form of the disease.

Plus, with British researchers from the University of Nottingham a step closer to developing a new blood test that detects cancer before it grows and before a tumour has had a chance to take shape, the National Cancer Intelligence Network may well have to revise their estimates. The test is the first to identify accurately the signals sent out by a person's immune system as a cancer germinates.

Research has shown that cancers involve irregular cells producing small amounts of protein material called antigens. These prompt the immune system to react, producing large amounts of auto-antibodies. By tracking this activity, and identifying which combination of antigens signals the presence of a particular cancer, scientists have been able to create a reproducible test which simply requires 10ml of blood from a patient. Respiratory specialists and family doctors in the US have been piloting the test on smokers. In many cases it either confirmed suspicions of a cancer, or prompted surgical intervention on a cancerous nodule previously thought to be benign *(Times online, 01/06/2010).*

With exciting developments like this, not to mention the cancer treatments listed in *The Cancer Survival Manual – Tomorrow's Cancer Breakthroughs TODAY* that have been scientifically proven to increase your chances of successfully battling the disease, the future looks very promising indeed.

Further reading

Living Proof: A Medical Mutiny by Michael Gearin-Tosh (Scribner; New edition edition). Michael Gearin-Tosh discovered that he had bone marrow cancer when he was 54. This is the story of his quest to manage and overcome his illness and his determination not to be coerced by specialists, the NHS and even colleagues into joining programmes of invasive treatments. The author selected a number of regimes and devised his own rigorous daily round of juices, vegetables and coffee enemas. This is an account of one man's quest to listen to his own inner voice of intuition in a world so heavily reliant on the certainty that it is the doctors that know best.

Waking the Warrior Goddess by Dr Christine Horner (Basic Health Publications). This book explores the various foods and supplements that can enable you to successfully fight breast cancer and claim the healthy body that should be yours. Using the metaphor of the Warrior Goddess, it explains something that Ayurveda describes as 'your inner healing intelligence'. Dr Horner tells you what to avoid and what to embrace, what will poison your Warrior Goddess and what will feed her what she needs to thrive.

Breast Cancer Survival Manual, Fourth Edition: A Step-By-Step Guide for the Woman with Newly Diagnosed Breast Cancer by Dr John Link (Owl Books). Includes the most current advice on: getting a second opinion, why it's important, what questions to ask, and how to decide which team of doctors is best for you; updates on genetic testing and how doctors are using the results to tailor care for each patient; and navigating new types of radiation, the Herceptin breakthrough, and improved reconstruction surgeries. Conscious of the rapidly evolving spectrum of treatment options, Dr John Link outlines the latest findings and professional wisdom for the patient in pursuit of the most effective treatment plan.

Prostate Cancer: Understand, Prevent and Overcome Prostrate Cancer by Professor Jane Plant (Virgin Books). Following the international success of *Your Life in Your Hands*, the ground-breaking book on breast cancer, Professor Jane Plant explains how her diet and lifestyle plan can be used to combat prostate cancer. This revised and updated edition includes new information to help those with other types of cancer, such as colorectal cancer and testicular cancer. In this book, Professor Plant illuminates the relationship between the disease and diet. The book explains the science behind the 'no dairy' diet and then gives useful advice on diet and lifestyle to maximise your health and avoid contracting cancer. For sufferers, their families and anyone who is concerned about the risk of cancer, this book is essential.

World Without Cancer: The Story of Vitamin B17, by G. Edward Griffin (American Media). Provides an excellent exposé of an alternative natural way to prevent and cure cancer through nutrition, and the forces in government and in large pharmaceutical firms that are fighting to keep the secret from us.

What to Eat if You Have Cancer (revised): Healing Foods that Boost Your Immune System by Maureen Keane (McGraw-Hill Contemporary). Cancer and cancer treatment take a toll on your body, but you can help make cancer treatment more effective and reduce its unpleasant side effects with good nutrition. *What to Eat if You Have Cancer* presents the best foods to fight cancer and suggests ways to keep your body strong. A vital resource for cancer patients, this revised edition contains new recipes, new menus, and the latest research on cancer and nutrition.

Healing the Gerson Way: Defeating Cancer and Other Chronic Diseases, by Charlotte Gerson and Beata Bishop. Gerson therapy is one of the metabolic therapies which uses a special diet, plus supplements, and a coffee enema to help the body heal itself and cure it of cancer.

A Time to Heal, by Beata Bishop. A truly inspirational book written by a former cancer patient, who recovered from metastasised malignant melanoma after following the Gerson therapy. Beata Bishop chose the therapy as a last resort in January 1981, when despite extensive surgery the melanoma had spread into her lymphatic system and orthodox oncology could only offer more surgery, without which her life expectancy was somewhere between six weeks and six months. Having thoroughly researched the disease Beata knew that further operations were not the answer, so embarked on the Gerson programme to try to rebuild her body's defences, so that it could eliminate the malignant process rather than weaken it further with radio or chemotherapy simply in order to shrink the tumour. After two tough years she was cured, and has remained so ever since.

Helpful organisations

Macmillan Cancer Support provides practical, medical and financial support and push for better cancer care. If you have any questions about cancer, need support or just someone to talk to, you can call free, Monday to Friday 9am-8pm (interpretation service available) – Tel: 0808 808 0000. Write to: Macmillan Cancer Support, 89 Albert Embankment, London SE1 7UQ. Visit: **www.macmillan.org.uk**

Cancer Research UK is the world's leading charity dedicated to beating cancer through research. Researches the causes, prevention and treatment of cancer. It also provides lots of information on cancer. Tel: 020 7242 0200; Visit: **www.cancerresearchuk.org**

Cancer Options is a private, cancer consultancy where you can obtain information on the different cancer treatments and therapies. You will find the best of orthodox and complementary approaches evaluated by Britain's leading experts in the integrative field. Cancer Options Ltd, PO Box 6778, Kirkby in Ashfield, Nottingham NG17 7QU, United Kingdom. Tel: 0845 009 204; Visit: **www.canceroptions.co.uk**

Hospice Information. Provide information to the public and professionals on hospice and palliative care in the UK and internationally. Tel: 020 7520 8222; Visit: **www.helpthehospices.org.uk/hospiceinformation**

Marie Curie Cancer Care. Marie Curie Nurses provide free nursing care to cancer patients and those with other terminal illnesses in their own homes. Marie Curie Nurses now care for around 50 per cent of all cancer patients who die at home. They work through the night or during the day to provide care for patients in the comfortable and familiar surroundings of their own home.

Marie Curie Cancer Care, 89 Albert Embankment, London SE1 7TP. Tel: 0800 716 146; Visit: **www.mariecurie.org.uk**

Cancer Chat. An online forum for people affected by cancer to share information and experiences, provided by Cancer Research. Visit: **www.cancerchat.org.uk**

The Prostate Cancer Charity is the UK's leading voluntary organisation working with people affected by prostate cancer. It provides the only UK-wide prostate cancer helpline staffed by prostate cancer specialist nurses who offer free and confidential information and support to anyone affected by prostate cancer. They also provide free information tailored to the needs of men with prostate cancer and their families. The Prostate Cancer Charity, First Floor, Cambridge House, 100 Cambridge Grove, Hammersmith, London W6 0LE. Freephone Helpline Number: 0800 074 8383 (Monday to Friday 10am - 4pm; plus late night Wednesday 7pm - 9pm). Calls are free of charge from UK landlines. Visit: **www.prostate-cancer.org.uk**

Prostate UK. Fund medical research, the training of healthcare professionals and provide information on all prostate diseases. Prostate UK, 6 Crescent Stables, 139 Upper Richmond Road, London SW15 2TN. Tel: 020 8788 7720; Visit: **www.prostateuk.org**

Breast Cancer care. Provide information and offer emotional and practical support to breast cancer sufferers and bring people affected by breast cancer together. Breast Cancer Care, 5-13 Great Suffolk Street, London SE1 0NS. If you have a specific enquiry about breast cancer or breast cancer treatment and are in the UK, you can call the freephone helpline on 0808 800 6000 (textphone 0808 800 6001) between 9am and 5pm, Monday to Friday, or between 9am and 2pm on Saturdays to speak to someone. Visit: **www.breastcancercare.org.uk**

Against Breast Cancer. Funds a research programme into new treatment and prevention of breast cancer. Researchers based at University College London Hospital aim to find a vaccine against breast cancer. They are looking at how the cancer cell, patients' natural resistance and environment (especially diet and lifestyle) interact. Tel: 01235 534 211; Visit: **www.aabc.org.uk**

Beating Bowel Cancer. Charity that provides information about all aspects of bowel cancer and provides a range of support services. Beating Bowel Cancer, Harlequin House, 7 High Street, Teddington TW11 8EE. Tel: 08450 719301; Visit: **www.beatingbowelcancer.org**

Bowel Cancer UK. Aims to sustain the normal quality of life, increase the cure rate and to prolong the survival of colorectal cancer patients. Bowel Cancer UK, 7 Rickett Street, London SW6 1RU. Tel: 020 7381 9711; Visit: **www.bowelcanceruk.org.uk**

Pancreatic Cancer UK. Charity that aims to give patients and their families access to the best possible support, information, treatment and care. Pancreatic Cancer UK, 3rd Floor, Market Towers, 1 Nine Elms Lane, London SW8 5NQ. Tel: 0203 177 1686; Visit: **www.pancreaticcancer.org.uk**

UCAN. Stands for Urological CANcers – a charity dedicated to raising awareness of urological cancers (including kidney, prostate, bladder and testicular cancers) and improving support and quality of life for people and families who are affected. Tel: (01224) 559312/553104; Visit: **www.ucanhelp.org.uk**

Jo's Cervical Cancer Trust (Jo's Trust) is the only UK charity dedicated to women and their families affected by cervical cancer and cervical abnormalities. Jo's Cervical Cancer Trust, 16 Lincoln's Inn Fields, London WC2A 3ED. Tel: 020 7936 7498; Visit: **www.jostrust.org.uk**

Ovarian Cancer Action is committed to improving survival for women with ovarian cancer through research, awareness and giving a voice. Tel: 0300 456 4700; Visit: **www.ovarian.org.uk**

British Lung Foundation is the only UK charity working for everyone affected by lung disease – from asthma to lung cancer. They support people affected by lung disease through the individual challenges they will face. British Lung Foundation, 73–75 Goswell Road, London EC1V 7ER. All letters are responded to within 4 working days. Visit: **www.lunguk.org;** Helpline Advice Service: 08458 50 50 20 (Mon to Fri 10 am to 6 pm)

The Gerson® Support Group UK (GSG) is a UK registered charity (no. 1063646). Founded by recovered cancer patients in 1993, it provides information, practical training and support to patients and their carers. The Gerson Therapy® is a holistic and natural treatment which utilizes the body's own healing mechanism in the treatment and cure of chronic, degenerative illness. There are plans to open a small day centre/drop in service in the UK soon (contact them for more details). Helpline: ((0)1372 464557), Visit: **www.gersonsupportgroup.org.uk**

Citizens Advice Bureaux. If you or a loved one is diagnosed with cancer, your local Citizens Advice Bureau can provide you with information on your rights as an employee if you require it. Visit: **www.citizensadvice.org.uk**

The British Association for Counselling and Psychotherapy, BACP House, 15 St John's Business Park, Lutterworth, Leics LE17 4HB. Tel: 01455 88 3300; Visit: **www.bacp.co.uk**

Institute for Complementary and Natural Medicine. Supplies names of practitioners of various kinds of complementary medicine. Tel: 020 7922 7980; Visit: **www.i-c-m.org.uk**

The Dove Clinic. The Dove Clinic, based in Twyford near Winchester and in Central London, offers alternative and complementary therapies for a wide range of illnesses and conditions, including cancer. London Clinic, 19 Wimpole Street, London W1G 8GE. Tel: 020 7580 8886; Visit: **www.doveclinic.com**

The British Association for Applied Nutrition and Nutritional Therapy, 27 Old Gloucester Street, London WC1N 3XX. Tel: 0870 606 1284; Visit: **www.bant.org.uk**

The Nutri Centre – the UK's leading supplier of vitamin and mineral supplements and herbal remedies. The Nutri Centre, 7 Park Crescent, London W1B 1PF; Tel: 0207 436 5122; Visit: **www.nutricentre.com**

Revital – online health store that supplies a wide range of nutritional supplements, health foods and herbal remedies. Revital Limited, Unit D3, Braintree Industrial Estate, Braintree Road, Ruislip, Middlesex HA4 0EJ. Tel: 0870 366 5729; Visit: **www.revital.co.uk**